T0205802

Mindful Medical Practitioners

Patricia Lynn Dobkin • Craig Stephen Hassed

Mindful Medical Practitioners

A Guide for Clinicians and Educators

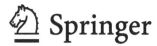 Springer

Patricia Lynn Dobkin
Faculty of Medicine, Programs in Whole
Person Care
McGill University
Montreal, QC
Canada

Craig Stephen Hassed
Monash University
Melbourne, VIC
Australia

ISBN 978-3-319-80954-0   ISBN 978-3-319-31066-4   (eBook)
DOI 10.1007/978-3-319-31066-4

Printed on acid-free paper

This Springer imprint is published by Springer Nature
The registered company is Springer International Publishing AG Switzerland

For Mark Smith, Gail Gauthier, Nancy Dobkin and my siblings: Sharon, Dennis, Sarah and Joseph – all who have encouraged me to live my Truth.

Dr. Patricia Lynn Dobkin

I dedicate this book to my wonderfully supportive colleagues at Monash University who have provided the space, encouragement and curriculum time to introduce mindfulness into the medical curriculum here. Just as a seed without fertile ground will not grow, without their open-mindedness and support this innovation would never have come to fruition.

Dr. Craig Stephen Hassed

Foreword

To do nothing is sometimes a good remedy.

Hippocrates

If you were living on the Peloponnesian peninsula in the fifth century B.C.E. and were in need of healing, and after having consulted local healers without improvement, you might make the arduous journey to one of the healing centres of the ancient world, such as the one in Epidaurus. There you would participate in community activities such as the gymnasium or theatre and eventually enter the Asclepeion temple for consultation with the priests and physicians. During this time period, as the Hippocratic approaches were demonstrating superior outcomes to other rational and non-rational healing modalities of the day, an integration of physical, psychological and spiritual information was used to effect healings that have been documented, much like the case records found in the *New England Journal of Medicine*, inscribed in stone for future generations to ponder the nature of illness, suffering and healing.

This was an exciting new era, ushering in the modern age of medicine, and with its successes was a developing pedagogy for passing along not just information but an approach and a world view to future generations. For Hippocrates, the physician and teacher role blended well when he started a school for medicine in Cos around 400 B.C. One of the main things that he taught was awareness and observation skills, and the importance of keeping a record through the observations of the patient's condition and symptoms. This honing of observation skills (which is not exactly to do nothing) through attention and awareness of the senses remains even today the primary means of data gathering for the health-care professional. In fact, every instrument in medicine that measures any parameter is literally an extension of the senses.

The modern era is an equally exciting and dynamic time for medicine, especially for health professional education. Advances in searching and retrieving clinically relevant information has extended beyond our imagination the capacity for an individual health-care professional to apply current evidence-based information to diagnose and heal. It is no longer necessary to master, through memorisation, reams of information much of which becomes obsolete over time. Rather, the emphasis of health professionals – physicians, nurses, therapists and others – can once again return to its patient-centred focus: to listen, to touch, to see and to use all the primary senses with the objective of developing a specific intimacy with the present health concerns, and through that relationship effect healing.

However, the inertia of over a hundred years of the current model of medical education makes it difficult to imbed, in a serious and meaningful way, educational approaches and objectives that promote self-care, self-awareness, empathy, compassion, contemplative practice, reflective practice and narrative analysis into curricula in the health-care professions. Dobkin and Hassed, in this highly readable and practical book, provide not only examples of where this is taking place in three different medical schools worldwide, but they provide a roadmap for a mindful approach to anyone interested in advancing mindfulness-based approaches in health-care professional education anywhere – mindful, because the discussion is based in reality, with an insightful and realistic assessment of the landscape in medical education; mindful, because the conversation invites an opening to the potentialities one can discover, wherever one finds oneself; and mindful, because the dialogue occurs right here, in the present moment, without judgment.

In a very clear, logical and methodical manner, the book opens with a discussion of the benefits that teaching Mindful Medical Practice have not only for students, patients and practising clinicians, but for the health-care system as a whole in terms of the quality of care and quality of caring it imparts. Building on this potential, it stresses the interdependent nature of self-care and the care of others and the role of mindfulness in further strengthening the argument for prominently featuring Mindful Medical Practice in medical education. Before describing three different examples of mindfulness in medical education, a thorough review of the evidence base for mindfulness in general, and more specifically, what is understood about its applications in medicine reveal its multi-faceted impact on of stress management, prevention of burnout, the cultivation of resilience and workplace engagement and meaning.

Rather than speak only about ideals, the discussion then proceeds with concrete examples of not only what is in place in specific medical educational institutions, but how these programs came into existence. This gives the reader an inside view of the cultural nuances, the creativity, the resistance and the acceptance met by innovators who worked skilfully at grass-roots and leadership levels to bring aspects of Mindful Medical Practice to students. While making a strong case for understanding on a deep personal level the qualities of mindfulness and how to most skilfully cultivate them, the reader is shown many different forms of expression, always remaining close to the qualities of beginner's mind, curiosity, acceptance, non-judgment and a trust in one's capacity to discover how best to deliver programs given many different local, cultural and historical topographies. Among the assets of this book, for the reader who is contemplating, introducing Mindful Medical Practice curricula into health-care professional education are the many examples of programs from far-flung places that demonstrate how committed health professionals and educators work together through the tasks of program delivery teacher training, individual and institutional resistance and prevailing cultural challenges.

The authors of *Mindful Medical Practitioners: A Guide for Clinicians and Educators* point out that Mindful Medical Practice is not a panacea for all that ails medical education. Yet, they create a cogent argument for how it can promote the kinds of leadership and cultural changes necessary to address many challenges facing health professionals. These include the well-being and longevity of physicians, nurses, therapists and others engaged in the care, ultimately, of all of us.

Not only will the medical educator from a variety of disciplines who is interested in mindfulness in health-care professional curricula find this book compelling, but so too will the student from many health professions discover the possibilities of including self-care and self-awareness as core competencies to develop through the educational continuum. Additionally, medical educational leadership at the under-graduate, graduate and professional/clinical levels will find in these pages insights about how to create a healthier and more resilient institutional culture.

Hippocrates was quoted as saying, 'It is more important to know what sort of person has a disease than to know what sort of disease has a person'. It may equally be more important to know what sort of health-care professional attends to the disease, than to know what sort of disease attends to the health professional. Thus it may be possible, through the development of a more self-aware, self-reflective and mindful medical practitioner, for healing to occur with the patient and the practitio-ner united in an exchange of caring that flows bidirectionally and includes attending to the self and to others. *Mindful Medical Practitioners: A Guide for Clinicians and Educators* points the way.

Michael Krasner, MD

Preface

Since the publication of Epstein's seminal paper in the *Journal of the American Medical Association* on Mindful Practice in 1999 [1], there has been a steady rise in the interest in mindfulness in general, and its application in clinical practice, in particular. Dobkin and Hutchinson summarised where and by whom mindfulness was being taught in medical schools in a review article published in Medical Education in 2013 [2]. This was followed by a series of related papers [3–8]. Model programs embedded in core curriculum have been offered at the University of Rochester School of Medicine and Dentistry by Epstein and his colleagues, as well as Hassed and his colleagues at Monash University Medical School in Australia [9]. Among other things, these undergraduate and postgraduate programs have demonstrated significant improvements in clinical and communication skills, empathy and various markers of well-being and study engagement [10, 11]. As a result of these publications, requests for conducting workshops, presentations at conferences, in hospital and academic settings and help setting up programs have increased from around the world. Mindful Medical Practice is becoming mainstream. For example, the Royal College of Physicians in Canada requires that psychiatry residents have some training (e.g. seminars) in mindfulness.

The programs offered and their formats, while often based on Mindfulness-Based Stress Reduction, vary considerably. This book is a logical follow-up on the Medical Education paper [2] and the authors' recent books, *Mindful Medical Practice: Clinical Narratives and Therapeutic Insights and Mindful Learning* [12, 13]. In particular, it aims not only to describe in more detail the ways mindfulness is being taught to medical students, residents, practising physicians and allied health-care professionals (e.g. psychologists, nurses), it also presents how programs are set up and integrated into curriculums. Our intention is to raise interest, inform, provide a rationale and address questions with regard to how to integrate mindfulness into clinical work, as well as be a guide and resource for those qualified to teach it.

Montreal, QC, Canada   Patricia Lynn Dobkin
Melbourne, VIC, Australia   Craig Stephen Hassed

References

1. Epstein R. Mindful practice. JAMA. 1999;282:833–9.
2. Dobkin PL, Hutchinson TA. Teaching mindfulness in medical school: where are we now and where are we going? Med Educ. 2013;47:768–79.
3. Hutchinson TA, Dobkin PL. Mindful medical practice: just another fad? Can Fam Phys. 2013;55(8):778–9.
4. Irving JA, Dobkin PL, Park J. Cultivating mindfulness in health care professionals: a review of empirical studies of Mindfulness-Based Stress Reduction (MBSR). Compliment Therap Clinic Practice. 2009;15(2):61–6.
5. Dobkin PL, Hutchinson TA. Primary prevention for future doctors: promoting well-being in trainees. Med Educ. 2010;44(3):224–6.
6. Garneau K, Hutchinson T, Zhao Q, Dobkin PL. Cultivating person-centered medicine in future physicians. Eur J Person-Centred Healthc. 2013;1(2):468–77.
7. Irving J, Park J, Fitzpatrick M, Dobkin PL, Chen A, Hutchinson T. Experiences of health care professionals enrolled in Mindfulness-Based Medical Practice: a grounded theory model. Mindfulness. 2014;5(1):60–71.
8. Dobkin PL, Laliberté V. Being a mindful clinical teacher: Can mindfulness enhance education in a clinical setting? Med Teacher. 2014;36(4):347–52.
9. Hassed C. Know thyself: the stress release programme. Australia: Michelle Anderson Publishing PTY Ltd; 2006.
10. Krasner MS, Epstein RM, Beckman H, Suchman AL, Chapman B, Mooney CJ, Quill TE. Association of an educational program in mindful communication with burnout, empathy, and attitudes among primary care physicians. JAMA. 2009;302(12):1284–93. doi: 10.1001/jama.2009.1384.
11. Hassed C, de Lisle S, Sullivan G, Pier C. Enhancing the health of medical students: outcomes of an integrated mindfulness and lifestyle program. Adv Health Sci Educ Theory Pract. 2009;14(3):387–98. doi: 10.1007/s10459-008-9125-3.
12. Dobkin PL, editor. Mindful medical practice: clinical narratives and therapeutic insights. Switzerland: Springer International Publishing; 2015.
13. Hassed C, Chambers R. Mindful learning. Sydney: Exisle; 2014.

Acknowledgments

A finished book stems from a series of events and exchanges that result in words strung together in sentences, which arrange themselves in paragraphs on pages, subdivide into chapters that aim to transmit what is in one mind (or two minds, in this case) to another. What inspires us to write a book is a different matter, for example, receiving requests and feedback such as these:

Hi Dr. Dobkin,

My name is Kareem and I'm a medical student at Vanderbilt University. I hope this message finds you well.

A few friends and I are planning to create a mindfulness elective for medical students here, and I saw online that you teach an elective called Mindful Medical Practice at McGill. I was wondering if you would be open to sharing your syllabus for the class and/or any other helpful resources or advice.

Take care,

Kareem

Hello Craig,

I had the great fortune to take your "Stress Management" elective in the First Year of my MBBS at Monash in 1994. It was extremely valuable and I find it still enables me to focus on the important things in life and at work (anaesthesia).

Kind regards,

Ian

The response to this and similar queries is this book. So first of all, we would like to acknowledge all of the people over the years who have asked, 'How can we start a program to teach mindfulness in our medical setting?'

Second, we would like to acknowledge the medical students, residents, physicians and allied health-care professionals who took our courses and participated in our workshops over the years; there are thousands of them. We have learned as much from them as they may have from us.

Third, we would like to acknowledge colleagues who have provided support and made this possible, first at McGill University, Dr. David Eidelman, the Dean of Medicine, and Dr. James Martin, the Physician-in-Chief who endorse our endeavours at McGill Programs in Whole Person Care; and second, at Monash University, Prof. Leon Piterman, Pro. Vice-Chancellor and former head of the Department of General Practice, and Sally Trembath and the Monash Mental Health Working Party who supported the creation of Mindfulness at Monash. We would also like to thank our colleagues who teach mindfulness at our medical schools: Drs. Tom Hutchinson, Stephen Liben and Mark Smilovitch have been key at McGill and Dr. Richard Chambers and a wonderful team of passionate and committed tutors at Monash; being part of these teams has been rich and rewarding. Ms. Angelica Todireau has been behind the scenes making sure all of our programs run smoothly at McGill. She was instrumental in completing this book from the first to last page.

Fourth, our colleagues at the University of Rochester School of Medicine and Dentistry, whose pioneering work is documented in this book, have always shared their know-how in a spirit of cooperation and collaboration.

Finally, there are people who have encouraged me (PLD) to write from child-hood (my late father, Robert D. Dobkin) through adulthood (my brother, Dr. Dennis Dobkin) and Mark S. Smith, my muse. And I (CH) would like to thank my wife, Deirdre, for all her love and unfailing support. Writing is essentially a solitary endeavour, but having people who believe in your aptitude is a blessing. Thus, we are grateful for their encouragement and support. Last but certainly not least, we wish to thank each other for being a pleasure to work with while 'finding one voice' in writing this book together. Collaboration doesn't happen without a shared vision and passion.

Contents

Chapter 1
Why Teach Mindfulness to Clinicians?

PreambleMourning Rounds

> 'Good morning', I said.
> 'Come closer', she asked.
> I usually did not, could not,
> standing in the doorway.
> 'Do you need anything?'
> 'Come closer', she said.
> 'I am close'. I thought.
> The room was small, filled by her bed.
> 'I mean near the bed – next to me – so I can see you.'
> I moved closer, foreseeing her death, which I could not prevent.
> 'I like it when you are close.'
> I moved even closer, reaching for her hand.
> 'That's what I really wanted
> – to touch your hand – to thank you.'
> She smiled, her face aglow,
> and I wept silently
> as I moved even closer
> to kiss her cheek
> to thank her
> for asking me to come closer
> when I thought I could not [1].

Who is this physician standing at the threshold of the patient's hospital room attending to her from what he perceives as a safe distance? When did he become more at ease extending words from the doorway rather than taking her hand at her bedside? Why did he not enter when asked to do so?

We offer here a hypothetical narrative about this physician who was once a medical student with an ardent desire to care for his fellow human beings.

On the morning of these Mourning Rounds, the physician rose at dawn, slipped into dark blue trousers, selected a light blue shirt, adjusted a silk tie and tiptoed out so as not to rouse his wife. He is a man who attends to details and his attire reflects that. In fact, all of his clothes were hung up colour coded so that he could dress

© Springer International Publishing Switzerland 2016
P.L. Dobkin, C.S. Hassed, *Mindful Medical Practitioners*,
DOI 10.1007/978-3-319-31066-4_1

without turning on the light. This ritual of leaving home and arriving at the hospital at 7 AM for rounds has been an integral part of his life for 35 years. Following a short drive to the hospital, he went to his office, donned a white coat, clipped his badge to the pocket and draped his stethoscope around his neck. He is a cardiologist and being a specialist gives him a sense of accomplishment and satisfaction. He aspired to be a doctor ever since he read the book *Great Expectations* when he was 12 years old. Having been born into a working man's family with immigrant grandparents, he was never prodded to become a physician. His colleagues would describe him as exceptionally competent, reliable, honest, hardworking and well read.

On the morning of these particular rounds, he was alert albeit somewhat tired – working into his 60s has taken its toll. Before reaching the doorway of the woman who requested his presence, he had reviewed the night shift events with the chief resident, checked in on several other patients, answered two pages and responded to a 45-year-old male admitted into the emergency department. All routine.

Nonetheless, many aspects of his work were taxing, not least of which were its unpredictability and dealing with uncertainty. Patients and their diseases could make demands at any time, and the best way forward is never as clear as it appears in textbooks. He could complete his weekend call schedule and drop into sleep only to have an ER nurse waken him abruptly. The physician would dutifully drive through the darkness back to the hospital. Another trying part of his job was related to how the health-care system had changed over time. With technological advances more attention is now paid to screens than patients. Paper work stole time from patient care.

Last year a younger friend and colleague died suddenly of a MI while on vacation. The cardiologist sometimes ponders his own heart because his partner placed a stent in one of his own coronary arteries a decade earlier. Yet, he tries to not dwell on this fact believing genetics alone were responsible; his paternal grandmother died of a MI at 58 and his father had bypass heart surgery at 73. The stress of his job and the need for self-care were not generally taken into consideration as denial can be common among doctors regarding their own health. After all, acknowledging the relationship between mind, emotions and the heart was a mysterious and less tangible world than that of pharmaceuticals and surgical procedures and one from which many doctors prefer to retreat.

By the time he stood in that doorway, he had more patients die under his watch than he could name. In the past he had attended their funerals but only rarely did so now. This woman, with her impending demise, was one more of many. Did facing her death force him to face his? His training in residency and medical school had failed to prepare him for this as it did for many of his colleagues [2]. While he remains a moral man, one guided by liberal values, his heart had gradually hardened. This had happened so insidiously that he was not conscious of it. Likely, as suggested by Shapiro [3], this loss of felt emotion began when he was a medical student, observing his teachers suppressing or denying theirs rather than allowing sadness, regret, confusion, surprise, appreciation and joy – the entire range of emotions – to serve as guides connecting them to patients in a meaningful way. This was one way, or so it seemed, to protect oneself from burnout.

Did *who* was in the bed influence his stance near the door? He had been her husband's physician before congestive heart disease and diabetes took him down. The physician resigned himself to such inevitable outcomes. He had learned Spanish in college, even brushed up on it later so that he could communicate with patients like them. Her request for closeness, a gentle hand in hers, was congruent with her culture where touching is part of loving life and others. When he kissed her cheek, his mind flooded with memories of his deceased father who, being of Ukrainian decent, affectionately kissed his family members on the mouth. They were wet, those kisses. Just like the tears. When he thanked her with this gesture, his heart softened and in that moment they could both feel healing taking place.

This narrative highlights some of the reasons why we should teach mindfulness to clinicians. In this chapter we will touch upon how mindfulness contributes to medical students', residents', physicians' and other clinicians' well-being. A more comprehensive review is provided in Chap. 2 where we also summarise how mindfulness contributes to clinical practice. In subsequent chapters we present how, when and where teaching Mindful Medical Practice can be carried out in a contextualised, effective and sustainable way.

1.1 Medical Students

Shapiro suggested some time ago that medical education can have the effect of reducing empathy and putting trainee doctors out of touch with their emotions and how to be at ease with them. This is often seen as a way of 'hardening' students for the demands of their future work and protecting them from vicarious stress or having emotions impair judgment. However, in response to declining empathy and increases in stress and distress among medical students [4], elective programmes that teach mindfulness have been offered and studied for two decades. As early as 1998, Shapiro and her colleagues examined outcomes for medical students who took the structured 8-week Mindfulness-Based Stress Reduction (MBSR) programme developed at the University of Massachusetts Medical School by Kabat-Zinn and his colleagues [5]. In the first randomised control trial reported [6], premed, first and second year medical students were assigned to either the MBSR or wait-list control group – the latter were crossed over once the wait period was over. The MBSR programme was enhanced with exercises designed to enhance listening skills and empathy. Results favoured those in the MBSR group in that there were decreases in psychological distress and increases on empathy and spiritual experiences. Similarly, a randomised clinical trial conducted by the same researchers [7] almost a decade later compared three groups: (1) 1-month mindfulness meditation (a brief version of the MBSR programme), (2) somatic relaxation training and (3) control. The two intervention groups showed reductions in psychological distress and increases in positive mood states compared to the control group, but the meditation group showed the best results for positive mood states, reduction in rumination and distractive thoughts.

Other medical schools reported similar results when students were taught mindfulness [8]. Rosenzweig et al. [9] used a prospective cohort study design with 140 second year medical students who took the MBSR programme over 10 weeks. A non-randomised control group who attended seminars on complementary medicine served as a comparison. Pre-post-MBSR changes showed improvements on mood disturbance at the end of the programme, while those in the control group worsened over time. Eighty-eight per cent of the students in the MBSR group rated mindfulness as helpful or very helpful.

These early programmes were delivered as electives, so it is possible that the students who attended may not be typical of the entire cohort. One of the authors (CH) had found great benefit in personally applying mindfulness over many years and felt motivated to provide such content for training doctors. In 2002 a mindfulness programme was integrated as an assessable part of core curriculum. A description of this work and the results of the programme are presented in Chap. 2 [10]. Subsequent studies have shown that the mindfulness component of this programme also increases study engagement across the rest of the medical curriculum [11].

In a relatively large Norwegian study that included medical and clinical psychology students in a randomised clinical trial of a slightly modified MBSR (shorter class times and home practice assignments), significant effects were found for those taking MBSR on mental distress, well-being and non-reactivity but not for school-related stress or burnout [12]. Improvements were more evident in women, but the study may have been underpowered as only 26 men took the MBSR course. Interestingly, class attendance and home practice served as moderators; students who were more engaged in the practice showed better outcomes.

While a consensus is emerging that students who practise mindfulness benefit from it, little is known about which aspects of these programmes are helpful for students. A randomised controlled trial in which medical students were simply requested to practise meditation daily at home with CDs for 8 weeks indicated that, compared to the control group, these students perceived stress to be reduced and had lower anxiety scores both at the end of the practice time and at 8 weeks post-intervention follow-up. Apparently even this stripped down version of mediation training can be useful. While this may seem surprising, a systematic review and meta-analysis of meditation programmes for psychological stress and well-being based on 47 trials with 3,515 participants [13] found a moderate level of evidence for improvements in anxiety, depression and pain.

1.2   Residents

Fifteen years ago while teaching fourth year medical students, one of the authors (PLD) heard a story that influenced her decision to bring mindfulness into medical practice despite many obstacles. While in training, a surgical resident's brother died. Naturally he desired to attend his funeral. When he requested a leave of absence, the resident was turned down because no one was willing to cover for him.

The room fell silent while we reflected on this sad turn of events. Then the students engaged in a discussion of: What should the resident have done (he did not attend the funeral)? What would you do? What kind of work environment and culture would deny a 2-day leave during a family crisis? Some said they had chosen a particular specialty (e.g. dermatology) so as to be able to live more 'normal' lives. More than a few were young women who wondered when and how they would start a family.

Reports of resident burnout and mental health issues are alarming and have serious consequences for their lives and medical practice [14]. Lebensohn et al. [15] conducted a longitudinal study of 172 family medicine residents and found that emotional exhaustion, depersonalization (two scales from the burnout measure), positive affect and life satisfaction deteriorated over the 2-year training period. Residents deemed to be 'at risk' had lower levels of emotional intelligence, gratitude and mindfulness.

While websites (outlined in Chap. 6) indicate that there are mindfulness-based programmes being offered to help them cope better with the high demands of this phase of their training, we could not find published studies regarding of the impact of teaching them mindfulness skills [16].

1.3 Physicians

We propose that the cardiologist depicted in the narrative is typical with regard to the types of stressors he was exposed to and his struggle with emotional distance. He was constrained by the medical culture that has little tolerance for 'weakness' (e.g. doctors often go to work when they are sick) or expressed emotion. He, like many others, had to deal with the inherent strains of practising medicine over decades in the context of a shifting health-care system. Poor attitudes towards self-care and personal development can be seen as being embedded in the medical culture. Indeed, there are increasing calls for doctors to acknowledge and respond to these needs as illustrated by this quote from a surgical journal. 'Research shows that stress without conflict resolution may lead to burnout, which can contribute to impaired technical performance, medical errors, physical and mental health problems, and even increase the risk of suicide. Therefore, it is crucial that surgeons, and the organizations that train and employ them, recognize the early signs of stress and burnout, adopt adaptive coping strategies, and maintain a culture wherein work-life balance and surgeon well-being are shared goals' [17].

There are numerous sources of stress for physicians; some are external, such as a heavy patient load, time pressure, interpersonal staff conflict, lack of autonomy in the work environment, record keeping requirements, potential for litigation and financial concerns (e.g. debt load following training, high costs for insurance and office operations). Some stressors are internal, such as personality characteristics (e.g. perfectionism, obsessive-compulsive traits), harsh self-judgment, poor emotional regulation and vicarious trauma. Interestingly, cultivating self-compassion is associated with greater well-being and an enhanced attitude to self-improvement, an ability to learn from mistakes and aim for positive role models [18].

The need to address these issues was recognised by Irving et al. [19] who, in 2009, concluded that mindfulness aided health-care professionals (medical and psychology students, nurses, doctors, social workers, among others) to cope with the challenges they face on a daily basis. In fact, studies from around the world substantiate these results. Marin-Asuero et al. [20] working with primary care physicians in Spain, Moody et al. [21] supporting paediatric oncologists in Israel and New York, Lovas et al. [22] training dentists in Canada and Krasner et al. [23] in the United States who offered a modified version of MBSR with primary care physicians – to name but a few – all point to the benefits of training physicians to be able to handle stress and their emotions better, as well as communicate with more awareness, and balance their work-personal lives. Importantly, follow-up data show that these benefits are proving to be lasting [19, 24].

1.4 Well Clinicians Promote Wellness and Healing in Their Patients

Epstein and Krasner [25] stress the importance of promoting physician resilience as a gateway to providing quality patient care. Self-awareness and self-monitoring are viewed as precursors to becoming resilient and clinically competent as well as enhancing communication. For example, one needs to notice the presence of bias or that negative emotions are arising or thoughts are confused before being able to deal with events effectively. Impaired doctors make over six times as many clinical and technical errors because of a lack of self-monitoring [26], but by recognising external and internal stressors before one reacts to them, the clinician can make discerning decisions with regard to the optimal course of action. By combining mindfulness with congruence, i.e. awareness of the self, the other and the context, we contend that physicians can foster healing and be healed in the process of their work [27].

Krasner et al. [23] not only found that primary physicians who took their year-long course felt better, but they also reported a positive impact on empathy and psychosocial beliefs (e.g. the importance of attending to the patient's narrative about illness) consistent with patient-centred care. Focus groups conducted with some of these participants revealed that the physicians' ability to be attentive and listen deeply to patients' concerns helped them to respond to patients' needs more effectively [28]. For example, one doctor said,

> As far as my patients go; I am much more curious, instead of resentful. So when I'm running behind and a patient comes in with, you know, some vague sort of complaint, I try to switch my mind... OK, try to be more curious about it and forget the emotions you are feeling, just be curious, and that has really helped.

Similarly, in another qualitative study of Mindfulness-Based Medical Practice for health-care professionals [29], half of whom were doctors, one participant said,

It's new territory for me in my everyday practice, and I think I am able to listen better to what people have to say because I am trying to really just be there as opposed to 'o.k. I have a role to play, I'm here to listen but I have to fix you'… And I noticed that when I have this experience that even if something difficult has happened there is a very empathetic interaction. I think I don't have a plan that I came in with and I just… I just was present and that worked, by itself.

1.5 Conclusion

Thus, we conclude this chapter with the proposal that teaching Mindful Medical Practice may result in a win-win-win situation such that clinicians and patients benefit, directly and indirectly. One would anticipate that the health-care system would also note benefits, such as fewer errors, reduced litigation, increases in patient adherence to medical recommendations and satisfaction, as well as a greater sense of meaning and community in those who choose to serve their fellow human beings with the three C's: care, competence and compassion.

References

1. Rogers AI. Mourning rounds. The Pharos/Winter [Internet]. 2006 [cited 4 Feb 2015]. Available from: http://themindfuldoctor.com/prescriptions_mourning_rounds.html.
2. Gawande A. Being mortal: medicine and what matters in the end. Canada: Doubleday; 2014.
3. Shapiro J. Does medical education promote professional alexithymia? A call for attending to the emotions of patients and self in medical training. Acad Med. 2011;86(3):326–32.
4. Dyrbye LN, West CP, Satele D, Boone S, et al. Burnout among U.S. medical students, residents, and early career physicians relative to the general U.S. population. Acad Med. 2014;89(3):443–51.
5. Kabat-Zinn J. Full catastrophe living: using the wisdom of your body and mind to face stress, pain, and illness. New York: Bantam Dell; 1990.
6. Shapiro S, Schwartz G, Bonner G. Effects of mindfulness-based stress reduction on medical and premedical students. J Behav Med. 1998;21(6):581–99.
7. Jain S, Shapiro SL, Swanick S, Roesch SC, Mills PJ, Bell I, et al. A randomized controlled trial of mindfulness meditation versus relaxation training: effects on distress, positive states of mind, rumination, and distraction. Ann Behav Med. 2007;33(1):11–21.
8. Dobkin PL, Hutchinson TA. Teaching mindfulness in medical school: where are we now and where are we going? Med Educ. 2013;47:768–79.
9. Rosenzweig S, Reibel DK, Greeson JM, Brainard GC, et al. Mindfulness-based stress reduction lowers psychological distress in medical students. Teach Learn Med. 2003;15(2):88–92.
10. Hassed C, de Lisle S, Sullivan G, Pier C. Enhancing the health of medical students: outcomes of an integrated mindfulness and lifestyle program. Adv Health Sci Educ. 2009;14:387–98.
11. Opie J, Chambers R, Hassed C, Clarke D. Data on Monash 2013 medical students' personality, mindfulness and wellbeing. 2015 (In preparation).
12. de Vibe M, Solhaug I, Tyssen R, Friborg O, Rosenvinge JH, Sørlie T, et al. Mindfulness training for stress management: a randomised controlled study of medical and psychology students. BMC Med Educ. 2013;13:107. doi:10.1186/1472-6920-13-107.

13. Goyal M, Singh S, Sibinga EMS, Gould NF, Rowland-Seymour A, Sharma R, et al. Meditation programs for psychological stress and well-being. A systematic review and meta-analysis. JAMA Intern Med. 2014;174(3):357–68. doi:10.1001/jamainternmed.2013.13018.
14. Schneider C, Palmer D, Holt C, Wissink T, Matthew S. A wellness curricular intervention for family medicine residents to reduce depression and burnout. J Altern Complement Med. 2014;20(5):A148–9. doi:10.1089/acm.2014.5399.
15. Lebensohn P, Dodds S, Brooks A, Cook P, Schneider C, Woytowicz J, et al. A longitudinal study of well-being, burnout and emotional intelligence in family medicine residents. J Altern Complement Med. 2014;20(5):A8. doi:10.1089/acm.2014.5017.
16. McCray LW, Cronholm PF, Bogner HR, et al. Resident physician burnout: is there hope? Fam Med. 2008;40(9):626–32.
17. Bittner JG, Khan Z, Babu M, Hamed O. Stress, burnout, and maladaptive coping: strategies for surgeon well-being. Bull Am Coll Surg. 2011;96(8):17–22.
18. Breines JG, Chen S. Self-compassion increases self-improvement motivation. Personal Soc Psychol Bull. Published online 29 May 2012;42:415–429. doi:10.1177/0146167212445599.
19. Irving J, Dobkin PL, Park J. Cultivating mindfulness in health care professionals: a review of empirical studies of mindfulness-based stress reduction (MBSR). Complement Ther Clin Pract. 2009;15(2):61–6. doi:10.1016/j.ctcp.2009.01.002.
20. Asuero AM, Queraltó JM, Pujol-Ribera E, Berenguera A, Rodriguez-Blanco T, Epstein RM. Effectiveness of a mindfulness education program in primary health care professionals: a pragmatic controlled trial. J Contin Educ Health Prof. 2014;34(1):4–12. doi:10.1002/chp.21211.
21. Moody K, Kramer D, Santizo RO, Magro L, Wyshogrod D, Ambrosio J, et al. Helping the helpers: mindfulness training for burnout in pediatric oncology – a pilot program. J Pediatr Oncol Nurs. 2013;30(5):275–84. doi:10.1177/1043454213504497.
22. Lovas JG, Lovas DA, Lovas PM. Mindfulness and professionalism in dentistry. J Dent Educ. 2008;72(9):998–1009.
23. Krasner MS, Epstein RM, Beckman H, Suchman AL, Chapman B, Mooney CJ, et al. Association of an educational program in mindful communication with burnout, empathy, and attitudes among primary care physicians. JAMA. 2009;302(12):1284–93. doi:10.1001/jama.2009.1384.
24. Fortney L, Luchterhand C, Zakletskaia L, Zgierska A, Rakel D. Abbreviated mindfulness intervention for job satisfaction, quality of life, and compassion in primary care clinicians: a pilot study. Ann Fam Med. 2013;11(5):412–20. doi:10.1370/afm.1511.
25. Epstein RM, Krasner MS. Physician resilience: what it means, why it matters, and how to promote it. Acad Med. 2013;88(3):301–3. doi:10.1097/ACM.0b013e318280cff0.
26. Fahrenkopf AM, Sectish TC, Barger LK, Sharek PJ, Lewin D, Chiang VW, et al. Rates of medication errors among depressed and burnt out residents: prospective cohort study. BMJ. 2008;336:488.
27. Hutchinson T, Dobkin P. Discover mindful congruence. Le Spécialiste. 2015;17(1):31–2.
28. Beckman HB, Wendland M, Mooney C, Krasner MS, Quill TE, Suchman AL, et al. The impact of a program in mindful communication on primary care physicians. Acad Med. 2012; 87:1–5.
29. Irving JA, Park-Saltzman J, Fitzpatrick M, Dobkin PL, Chen A, Hutchinson T. Experiences of health care professionals enrolled in mindfulness-based medical practice: a grounded theory model. Mindfulness. 2014;5:60–71.

Chapter 2
Scientific Underpinnings and Evidence Pertaining to Mindfulness

2.1 Introduction

It is worth noting at the outset of this chapter that the principles and practices associated with mindfulness have been applied within many of the world's great spiritual or wisdom traditions for millennia, most notably in Buddhism. In the ancient world, they did not conduct clinical trials to guide practice. What they drew from was the evidence born of direct experience powered by a deep longing for self-knowledge, an acute spirit of inquiry and astute powers of observation. This evidence is important in and of itself and should not be ignored, but in the modern day, it is not sufficient to satisfy clinicians, scientists, educators and policy makers. Ultimately, this direct, experiential evidence is what has inspired and guided many of today's leading mindfulness practitioners and researchers. But the uptake of mindfulness needs to be seen within the scientific paradigm where personal experience and reflection is largely ignored by the majority of biomedically orientated scientists and where faith is mistrusted and evidence is highly valued.

It is doubtful that mindfulness would be widely known if it had not been for the explosion of research in the field since the early 2000s. For example, in the year 2000, there were seven new mindfulness citations on PubMed. In 2005, there were 31; in 2010, there were 190; and in 2015, there were 592 (as of September 20, 2015). The single biggest catalyst for this flurry of research activity was probably the evidence for mindfulness significantly reducing the likelihood of relapse for depression in those with multiple previous episodes. This arose from the work of John Teasdale, Mark Williams and Zindel Segal who took the principles of MBSR laid out by Jon Kabat-Zinn and developed Mindfulness-Based Cognitive Therapy (MBCT). Considering the looming burden of disease associated with depression, it is understandable that these benefits of mindfulness would stimulate keen interest. This gave a great deal of impetus to the work on the neuroscience of mindfulness which rapidly took off with researchers such as Sarah Lazar, Richard Davidson and Britta Holzel leading the way.

© Springer International Publishing Switzerland 2016
P.L. Dobkin, C.S. Hassed, *Mindful Medical Practitioners*,
DOI 10.1007/978-3-319-31066-4_2

Since then, the application of mindfulness to an incredibly wide range of areas has been documented. In some areas, the evidence base is becoming well established, whereas in others, it is still emerging. Although this could be the subject of an entire book, this chapter highlights fields of mindfulness research that are pertinent to medical education.

2.2 Overview of Mindfulness Research

Evidence for the application of mindfulness is well developed for preventing the relapse of depression. Studies vary in terms of their sample size and rigour, but, taken together, there is a clear picture developing of efficacy and applicability of mindfulness in selected areas, such as in the management of chronic pain and chronic illnesses.

In other fields such as attention deficit hyperactivity disorder or autistic spectrum, the evidence is limited to a small number of promising trials. While there is a sound rationale for its applicability, evidence is lacking to support widespread clinical uptake. Caution needs to be taken in all areas of mindfulness research, as it does in medicine more generally, so that unbridled enthusiasm for mindfulness doesn't exceed its efficacy or safe application. Prudence is also needed in the interpretation of mindfulness research. For example, a false-positive finding can be due to poor study design or biased interpretation of the data. Equally, false-negative findings may not be because mindfulness is not efficacious but result from small sample sizes, inadequate mindfulness instruction, incorrect application or misconstrued findings.

The areas of mindfulness research reviewed herein will be subdivided into a number of headings. We will emphasise the areas of research interest that are most relevant to medical students or clinicians either because they are important for their patients' or their own needs.

2.2.1 Clinical Performance and Decision-Making

The most influential person in this field has been Ronald Epstein from Rochester School of Medicine and Dentistry in the United States who put Mindful Practice on the map in 1999 [1]. Mindfulness can be viewed as a high-level clinical skill that should be taught in the undergraduate and postgraduate training of health practitioners. Some of the reasons for this will be briefly explored.

2.2.1.1 Executive Functioning

The prefrontal cortex contains most of the brain's important centres for executive functioning. Executive functions (EF) include:

- Attention regulation
- Self-awareness

- Working (short-term) memory
- Reasoning and decision-making
- Emotional regulation
- Appetite regulation
- Impulse control

The most essential EF could be seen as attention regulation because it is a prerequisite for the others. Without attention we cannot do anything else particularly well. This is because the attentional network is like a relay station for the other centres. If the attention doesn't engage, then the other centres won't either. So, for example, if we are inattentive, then working memory doesn't operate effectively and self-awareness – vital for introspection and insight – will not operate effectively either. If we are unaware, emotional regulation is difficult and resembles, at best, emotional suppression. Essential in emotional regulation is the ability to recognise, but not be caught up by emotions, through non-attachment to them. This makes it easier to express them in a more discerning way. A practitioner cannot function effectively without EF working well, and this links with a range of core clinical competencies.

2.2.1.2 Mindful Practice and Self-Monitoring

Epstein et al. stated, 'Mindful practice is conscious and intentional attentiveness to the present situation – the raw sensations, thoughts, and emotions as well as the interpretations, judgments and heuristics that one applies to a particular situation [2]'. Mindfulness contributes to self-monitoring, reducing errors, avoiding automatic pilot-type reactivity and establishing therapeutic relationships [3].

2.2.1.3 Cognitive Bias

Considerable work has uncovered reasons why clinicians make diagnostic errors. These are defined as misreading a clinical situation where the correct conclusion should have been evident from the clinical data. One explanation for bias is that it is cause d by the unconscious assumptions taken into clinical interactions. The two main forms of bias are:

- Confirmation bias: the pursuit of data that support a diagnosis over data that refute it
- Anchoring bias: a resistance to adapting appropriately to subsequent data that suggest alternative diagnoses [4]

The rationale for mindfulness is that the self-aware clinician is more likely to notice cognitive bias as it arises and will therefore be less influenced by it and less likely to mistake an assumption to be a fact. However, individual factors like cognitive bias should not be taken in isolation from the systemic factors that make them more likely to occur such as time pressure, fatigue, overwork and a distracting environment [5].

The case for mindfulness is largely drawn from the wider literature on attention and cognitive functioning and medical errors, but there is relatively little direct evidence measuring a reduction in diagnostic and clinical errors through the introduction of a mindfulness intervention. That, no doubt, will be another field of research to come.

2.2.1.4 Attention Deficit Trait and Multitasking

The modern world and attempts to adapt to its demands may be detrimental for maintaining attention. A newly recognised neurological phenomenon has been described by Hallowell and is termed 'attention deficit trait' (ADT). This is seen as a response to the hyperkinetic environment so much a part of modern professional life [6]. In such an environment, we find ourselves trying to deal with too much input which results in black-and-white thinking, difficulty staying organised, setting priorities, managing time and a constant feeling of low level of panic and guilt.

One of the ways we try to offset for such an environment is to multitask; this is defined as trying to pay attention to multiple complex tasks not serially but *at the same time*. This not only increases stress levels but unfortunately also increases errors and reduces performance. For example, driving while talking on a cellular phone is associated with over a fourfold increased likelihood of crashing, about the same impact as a 0.08 blood alcohol level [7]. Through multitasking, we compound the problem of demanding environments rather than alleviate it, whereas 'unitasking' with efficient attention switching is a valuable skill for dealing with such environments.

One of the greatest boons of contemporary living, and one of the greatest challenges, is the use and overuse of technology such as smartphones. These increase the likelihood of multitasking and distraction. A study of university students found that initially the utility of the smartphone to help with education was perceived as favourable, but by the end of the study, they viewed their phones as having a negative effect. The average response at the beginning of the first year of university education was 3.71 on a 1–5 scale (with one being 'strongly disagree' and five being 'strongly agree'). It dropped to 1.54 by the end of the year. When asked to rate the statement, 'My iPhone will distract/has distracted me from school-related tasks', the average response rose from 1.91 at the beginning of the study to 4.03 afterwards [8]. This is relevant for medical students, residents and clinicians who use their cellular phones throughout their waking hours every day of the week.

It is not just multitasking that negatively influences performance. There is also the impact of being in an environment where there are constant stimuli drawing the attention off-task. For example, one study of university students found that creating a distraction like the phone going off on vibration while performing another task was enough to increase the error rate by 28 % even if the student didn't answer it. Those who received a text were 23 % more likely to err [9]. Studies examining the effect of pager and phone alerts on clinical performance and error rates have not yet been conducted, but it is reasonable to expect similar results. Such evidence implies the need to train doctors to better micromanage attention in challenging clinical environments.

2.2.1.5 Vicarious Stress

Vicarious stress – being affected by another's distress – involves activation of limbic brain regions such as the amygdala and is implicated in empathic responses to another's suffering. When significant and prolonged, vicarious stress can lead to caregiver and compassion fatigue, burnout (depersonalisation), and impaired empathy. On the other hand, the ability to feel compassion and empathy without distress is increased with meditation and can reduce vicarious stress and caregiver fatigue. This is indicated in self-report and brain scans showing less activation of the amygdala but greater activation of brain regions associated with compassion while in the presence of another person's distress [10, 11].

More recently, studies have differentiated between neural changes associated with focussed attention meditation (FAM) and compassion or loving-kindness meditation (LKM) where a person attends to thoughts of kindness and compassion [12]. While only FAM enhanced performance on attentional tasks, FAM and LKM practices affected the neural responses to pictures designed to elicit an emotional response. For example, when viewing sad faces, the regions activated for FAM practitioners were consistent with attention-related processing, but responses of experts in LKM indicated an ability to differentiate 'emotional contagion' from the compassion/emotional regulation processes, i.e. they were able to experience compassion even in the presence of negative affect rather than being overwhelmed by it. This indicates that there may be two specific abilities that need development through meditation training. The development of compassion for others rests on the ability to be compassionate with oneself first.

2.2.1.6 Emotional Intelligence, Empathy and Communication

Mindfulness training has been found to increase physicians' ability to communicate with sensitivity and empathy with their patients as well as colleagues [13]. Observational studies of clinicians have compared clinicians with highest and lowest mindfulness scores [14]. High-mindfulness clinician consultations demonstrate:

- Patient-centred patterns of communication
- More rapport building and discussion of psychosocial issues
- More positive emotional tone with patients
- Patients more likely to give high ratings on clinician communication and to report high overall satisfaction

Rather than base findings on cross-sectional data, Dobkin et al. [15] conducted a prospective study with 25 clinicians (13 of whom were physicians) in Paris who were enrolled in an MBSR course. The physicians were tape-recorded while with the same patient before and after the program, and all patients rated the medical encounter pre- and post-MBSR using the Rochester Communication Rating Scale (RCRS). The audiotapes were coded by an independent team. Patients' independent ratings at the end of the study indicated increases in their clinicians':

- Interest in the patient as a person
- Understanding the patient's experience of illness
- Attention to context

There were significant improvements in clinicians' stress, and two burnout scales (depersonalisation and personal accomplishment), life being viewed as meaningful and mindfulness. Notably, decreased depersonalisation was significantly associated with the RCRS subscale, 'understanding the patient's experience of illness'.

Decreased clinician stress was significantly associated with three facets of mindfulness:

- Acting with awareness
- Non-reactivity
- Non-judgment

The audiotape data revealed a significant increase in 'backchannelling', i.e. indicating sustained interest (e.g. 'Go on…'). Backchannelling does not imply agreement or acceptance of ideas being expressed; rather, it reflects attentiveness. While the audiotape data appeared to show agreement and mutual understanding between the doctors and their patients increased over time, these findings are based on a small sample size and require replication.

The book *Mindful Medical Practice*: *Clinical Narratives and Therapeutic Insights* shows through the lens of 26 clinicians (mostly physicians) how mindfulness enhances their relationships with their patients and renders their work more meaningful [16].

2.2.2 Practitioner and Student Well-Being

2.2.2.1 Practitioner Mental Health and Burnout

As mentioned in Chap. 1, it has been well known for decades that medical professionals have far poorer health in certain areas than comparable demographic groups in the general community; these are depression and anxiety and higher rates of substance abuse. Developing resilience, a preventive approach to self-care, and early interventions are therefore essential to the education of medical students and doctors in training.

Willcock et al. [17] followed the mental health and burnout rates of new medical graduates from their final year and throughout their first year of work as interns. The results of this unique longitudinal study were alarming. By mid-final year, 28 % of medical students qualified as experiencing burnout; even worse, by 8 months into internship, 75 % interns qualified as experiencing burnout and 73 % met criteria for psychiatric morbidity on at least one occasion that year. It was the rule, not the exception, to report mental illness. This points to a major deficiency in how medical professionals are trained to carry out a demanding job where high expectations and standards are the norm, where concerns about the risk of errors and high workload are real in an environment characterised by low support and job control.

Work stress is not confined to the hospital setting. Resilience refers to an ability to cope with stress and adversity or to face, rise above and learn from difficult experiences. A survey of general practitioner postgraduate trainees by Cooke et al. [18] found that risk factors for burnout were secondary traumatic stress, intolerance of uncertainty, anxiety due to clinical uncertainty and reluctance to disclose uncertainty to patients. Only 10 % of trainees had high resilience scores; resilience was positively associated with compassion, satisfaction and personal meaning in patient care. Resilience was negatively associated with burnout, secondary traumatic stress, inhibitory anxiety, general intolerance to uncertainty, concern about bad outcomes and reluctance to disclose uncertainty to patients. Being comfortable with uncertainty, anxiety and discomfort, cultivating compassion for oneself and others are core attributes associated with mindfulness and have led to the call for mindfulness-based interventions to enhance physician resilience [19].

Another hidden cost of burnout is that it is associated with a significantly higher likelihood of unprofessional behaviours, less altruistic professional values, absenteeism, medical errors and suboptimal patient care [20]. One British Medical Journal study by Fahrenkopf et al. [21] estimated that a depressed resident makes more than six times as many medication errors as a nondepressed resident doing the same job. This is a strong argument for self-care to be seen as an investment in the well-being of the doctor and the patients they treat.

There is little use in listing problems without exploring solutions. A significant body of data suggests that various interventions can be effective for enhancing clinician well-being. One meta-analysis examined the effectiveness of interventions for stress, anxiety and burnout in physicians and medical trainees [22]. It was found that cognitive, behavioural and mindfulness-based interventions were associated with decreased symptoms of anxiety in physicians and medical students and that psycho-education, enhancing skills in interpersonal communication and mindfulness-based interventions were associated with decreased burnout in physicians.

To illustrate, a randomised clinical trial of practicing physicians in the United States compared with non-trial control participants explored the effect of an intervention consisting of 19 biweekly, facilitated physician discussion groups [23]. These groups incorporated elements of mindfulness, reflection, shared experience and small-group learning. The findings were that empowerment and engagement at work increased significantly in the intervention group versus a decline in the control group. This improvement was evident by 3 months and was sustained at 12 months. Rates of high depersonalisation, i.e. when patients are treated impersonally, had decreased at 3 months by 15.5 % in the intervention group versus a 0.8 % increase in the control group. Furthermore, the proportion of participants strongly agreed that their work was meaningful (this increased by 6.3 % in the study intervention group but decreased by 6.3 % in the control group and by 13.4 % in the non-study cohort over the study period). Rates of depersonalisation, emotional exhaustion and overall burnout also decreased substantially in the intervention group, decreased slightly in the control group and increased in the control group.

An 8-week mindfulness program (with monthly follow-up classes for a year) for primary care physicians by Krasner et al. showed improvements on all measures of well-being and clinical performance including:

- Reduced burnout
- Greater empathy and responsiveness to psychosocial aspects
- Less total mood disturbance
- Greater conscientiousness and engagement at work
- More emotional stability [24]

The improvements in mindfulness correlated with improvements on the other scales indicating that they were related to being more mindful. Another study on mindfulness training for clinicians found the magnitude of the positive change was large in total mood disturbance and mindfulness along with moderate improvements on burnout and empathy scores [25].

Irving et al. [26] conducted focus groups with a mixed group of health-care professionals (half of whom were physicians). Participants reported that when they completed the Mindfulness-Based Medical Practice course, they were more aware of cognitions, sensations and emotions that contributed to interpersonal patterns and dynamics. When they noticed their minds wandered, they were able to refocus. The regular practice of meditation enabled them to be more open-minded and compassionate towards themselves and others (including their patients). The clinicians were better able to regulate their emotions by focusing on the breath in stressful situations, and they were able to circumvent acting impulsively or automatically. This led them to see they had choices in how to respond.

In working with medical students at McGill University Medical School, we have found similar results even though the Mindful Medical Practice elective was fit into a month-long (rather than 8 week) time slot. Garneau et al. [27] reported that 58 fourth year medical students experienced decreased burnout, depression and stress as well as increased well-being, self-compassion and mindfulness after taking the course. Garneau described how he was able to maintain these benefits well into his family medicine residency. He wrote, 'Now, whenever I feel overwhelmed I make a conscious effort to listen to what my body is telling me. I learned to work within my limitations and take a step back when needed. I am more attentive, self-aware, curious and care more about my patients and myself as a result' [27] (p 474).

Note that Kevin Garneau included himself in who he took care of. Self-compassion is an important hallmark of a shift to a more mindful attitude towards oneself and is reflected in a changing attitude to others. Research has shown that self-compassion is associated with:

- Greater belief that a personal weakness can be changed for the better
- Greater motivation to make amends and avoid repeating a moral transgression

- More time studying for a difficult test following an initial failure
- A preference for upward social comparison after reflecting on a personal weakness
- Greater motivation to change the weakness [28]

There is no hard and fast answer to the question as to how much mindfulness meditation practice is necessary. Evidently the longer and more consistent the practice, the greater the progress in cultivating mindfulness. The 40 min per day recommended from the original research on MBSR and MBCT is probably a useful guide. One MBCT-based study found that people recovering from depression had half the relapse rate if they practiced meditation three or more times a week compared to less than three times a week [29]. Busy students and doctors, particularly if they have not self-selected to participate in a mindfulness course, or patients with lesser levels of distress may not be motivated to practice that much meditation. Interestingly, significant improvements have been found for psychological well-being [30], emotional regulation [31], reduced amygdala activation [32], pain tolerance [33] and cognitive functioning [34, 35] even with brief interventions and shorter durations of practice for non-clinical populations.

All medical students at Monash University have a mindfulness-based lifestyle and well-being program as a part of core curriculum. A study of these students found that over 90 % of them personally applied the mindfulness and lifestyle strategies by the end of the program and that correlated with improved student well-being on all measures even in the high-stress pre-exam period. Students were encouraged to practice mindfulness meditation for 5 min twice a day, but the majority only practiced a few times a week. The improvements, however, included reduced depression and anxiety, improved psychological and physical quality of life [36]. More recent studies on the Monash University cohort have confirmed that mindfulness training is associated with lower levels of distress and enhanced self-care [37]. This program will be described in more detail in Chap. 4. Another program developed by a former Monash tutor for the University of Tasmania medical course has shown similar findings [38]. Medical students who have been taught mindfulness and its clinical applications are far more likely to be disposed to recommend it to their patients one day [39].

2.2.3   *Learning and Academic Performance*

Reviews of the impact of mindfulness in educational settings do not address variability in study designs or their rigour. One review on academic performance concluded between-group effect sizes were largest for cognitive performance, stress and resilience [40]. To date, there are no studies testing whether mindfulness training increases student grades or prevents failure. There is, however, a rationale for how mindfulness may help student academic performance.

In order to understand how mindfulness might improve academic performance, it is important to consider factors that can impair it. Anxiety impairs executive functioning and leads to a smaller working memory [41]. 'Performance pressure harms individuals most qualified to succeed by consuming the working memory capacity that they rely on for their superior performance' [42]. Similarly, default mode, the state of mind we go into when distracted and inattentive, is also associated with poorer memory and executive functioning. These problems are present in various forms of psychopathology including depression, anxiety, schizophrenia and autism. Mindfulness has been found to improve student working memory and performance on attention tasks [43]. In three studies that examined the effects of mindfulness meditation on the knowledge retention those students who had practiced meditation briefly prior to a post-lecture quiz had improved retention of the information conveyed during the lecture compared to students who simply rested prior to the class [35].

Mindfulness has also been found to lead to reduced cognitive rigidity via the tendency to be 'blinded' by experience through 'a reduced tendency to overlook novel and adaptive ways of responding due to past experience, both in and out of the clinical setting'. In short, it aided participants to be more flexible problem solvers [44].

Another study on the Monash medical school cohort revealed that greater adherence to the mindfulness component of their medical course was associated with greater study engagement across the medical curriculum [45].

Although there is evidence of mindfulness improving cognitive functioning and working memory, the inferences of this translating into improved academic performance has been slower in coming. There has been a demonstrated reduction of anxiety and improved performance of students on high-stakes exams through the application of mindfulness training [46].

It is just as important for teachers to be as mindful as their students [47]. A randomised clinical trial of pilot program of Mindfulness-Based Stress Reduction adapted for teachers showed significant reductions in psychological symptoms and burnout, improvements in observer-rated classroom organisation and performance on a computer task of affective attentional bias and increases in self-compassion. The control group showed worse cortisol levels and increased burnout [48].

2.2.4 Neuroscience and Meditation

Contrary to decades of medical dogma, it is now known that the brain is continually wiring and rewiring itself throughout life according to what we think, how we behave and the environments we are in. This is neuroplasticity, and it begins to explain how we can unwire unhelpful patterns of thought and behaviour and wire in more adaptive ones. It is also now known that the adult brain has the capacity for neurogenesis, i.e. the ability to make new neurons. Mindfulness is at the forefront of this research.

Advances in brain imaging such as the use of MRI ad fMRI have made a significant difference in our ability to understand the immediate and long-term effects of mindfulness on the structure and function of the brain. There are books dedicated to this field, e.g. *The Mindful Brain* [49], *The Brain that Changes Itself* [50] and *Mindfulness and the Brain* [51]. There are also a number of reviews in major journals

[52]. For example, a paper in Nature Reviews Neuroscience [53] identified 21 studies demonstrating changes in brain structure and/or cortical thickness associated with the practice of mindfulness. In summary, they found changes in these brain regions:

- Frontopolar cortex associated with enhanced meta-awareness
- Sensory cortex and insula related to body awareness
- Hippocampus related to memory
- Anterior cingulate cortex, mid-cingulate cortex and orbitofrontal cortex related to self-awareness and emotional regulation
- Superior longitudinal fasciculus and corpus callosum involved with intra and inter-hemisphere communication

Mindfulness is associated with beneficial changes in the brain functioning in areas responsible for executive functioning, including attentional control, self-regulation as well as sensory processing, memory and regulation of the stress response [52, 54, 55]. There is an increase in grey matter density and thickness in regions associated with attention, self-awareness and sensory processing and memory [56] which is like reversing the assumed cortical thinning associated with ageing [57] indicating the 'neuroprotective effects and reduce the cognitive decline associated with normal ageing' [58].

Attentional states and the nature of leisure activity are also associated with long-term brain ageing and the risk of dementia. For example, older people who have greater participation in cognitively stimulating activities that involve learning, engagement, creativity and interaction (i.e. that demand attention) particularly in early and middle life activities have brains comparable to young people as indicated by reduced amyloid uptake. The elderly with the lowest levels of cognitive activity had brain changes comparable to patients with AD [59]. Predominantly passive leisure activities like television watching compared to active and engaging leisure activities throughout adult years are associated with nearly four times the likelihood of developing dementia [60, 61].

Mental illnesses like depression increase the risk of AD because of the secretion of high levels of neurotoxic cortisol and pro-inflammatory cytokines associated with overactivation of the sympathetic nervous system (allostatic load) in unhealthy emotional states and have been shown to cause thinning of grey matter particularly in the prefrontal cortex and hippocampus [62]. Regular practice of the 'relaxation response' (which differs from meditation) has been found to downregulate activation of the sympathetic nervous system and allostatic load [63].

The brains of adolescents brought up in hostile and unsupportive environments are predisposed to reproduce anti-social behaviours, attentional problems and learning difficulties in later life. This is largely related to overstimulation of the amygdala and underdevelopment of the prefrontal cortex [64–66] and is a particular problem for young men [67]. Mindfulness, on the other hand, has been shown to produce positive changes the opposite of these [68–71].

When not mindful, the brain switches into what is called 'default mode' characterised by distracted mental activity such as internal dialogue, daydreaming, reliving the past and projecting into the future. It expresses itself in various ways including depressive rumination and worry. Default mental activity in states of stress, anxiety and depression is plentiful and may partially explain why poor mental health is associated with loss of focus, self-referential thinking, and poor functioning [72]. Increased default mode or default mental activity may explain why doctors communicate more poorly, make more errors and have poorer memory when they are in such a mode. Unbridled default mode may have a long-term deleterious effect on the brain and has been associated with higher β-amyloid deposition leading on to a greater risk of Alzheimer's disease [73].

Mindfulness training switches on attentional and sensory networks and switches off the default network. Experienced practitioners are more able to do this because brain regions associated with self-monitoring and cognitive control respond much more quickly in them than in those less experienced in mindfulness [74]. They also have greater levels of connectivity between default and the executive functioning circuits meant to regulate it [75]. This has important implications for mental health, anxiety and the prevention of relapse into depression.

Although the full therapeutic and functional potential of mindfulness training is unknown, long-accepted medical doctrine is being challenged, and new potential therapeutic and self-development avenues are opening up.

2.2.5 Patient Health

2.2.5.1 Mental Health

For millennia, mindfulness-based approaches have been used as a means for reliving suffering. In the modern day, we call 'suffering' by different names like depression, stress and anxiety. Currently mindfulness is a foundation for various forms of psychotherapy. As the evidence base matures, questions over how large the effect sizes are and for whom it is most effective will be addressed [76].

The early studies on MBCT found that it halved the relapse rate for people who have had recurrent depression compared to treatment as usual [77]. MBCT reduces relapse rates by changing the relationship to negative and ruminative thoughts and emotions rather than by changing the belief in thought content itself, as is the case with conventional cognitive therapy [78]. Brain imaging indicates that changes in brain function during mindfulness include increased signals in regions related to mood regulation and attention control as well as an increased release of dopamine associated with positive mood states [71, 79]. Mindfulness reduces levels of inflammatory cytokines that cause the 'sickness response' and explains a range of symptoms associated with depression like lack of appetite, motivation and energy [80]. Mindfulness training reduces the reactivity of the amygdala, which is overactive in people with stress, anxiety and depression [81].

In adolescents, mindfulness reduces symptoms of anxiety, depression and somatic distress and increases self-esteem and sleep quality [82] with improved sleep likely one of the most important reasons why mindfulness is therapeutic for depression. The limited research available suggests that mindfulness improves sleep quality, sleep latency, sleep duration and the use of sleep medications [83]. Enhanced sleep may be part of the explanation for mindfulness reducing depression in those with chronic insomnia [84].

Mindfulness also helps with generalised anxiety and related symptoms (e.g. social anxiety disorder) [85] although it is not yet known if it is more effective than other previously studied approaches such as medications and Cognitive Behaviour Therapy [86].

Mindfulness-based strategies have been applied to people with schizophrenia who are in remission, with some promising results in terms of anxiety or being less intruded upon by residual symptoms [87, 88]. Mindfulness should be included in interventions for these disorders by mental health professionals experienced with mindfulness approaches and should be employed with caution for people with a past history of psychosis [89]. Intensive practice should also be avoided because of the potential to trigger psychotic episode. This approach for schizophrenia should not be seen as an alternative to medications.

MBSR has been found to produce improvement in self-reported post-traumatic stress disorder (PTSD) symptom severity during treatment and at 2-month follow-up with the MBSR group more likely to show clinically significant improvement in self-reported PTSD symptom severity (48.9 % versus 28.1 %) – loss of PTSD diagnosis (53.3 % versus 47.3 %) at 2-month follow-up [90]. Adult survivors of childhood sexual abuse who participated in an 8-week MBSR plus three refresher classes had depressive symptoms reduced by 65 % at the completion of the course and significant improvements in all outcomes (mood, anxiety, PTSD) post-MBSR and at 24-week follow-up [91]. Of three PTSD symptom criteria, symptoms of avoidance and numbing were most greatly reduced.

Mindfulness helps in the management of eating disorders by increasing awareness of the behavioural and physical cues, helping to deal with self-criticism and negative self-image and assisting in managing impulsivity and the negative emotions that are a common part of eating disorders [92]. Mindfulness programs for binge eating are designed to address:

- Controlling responses to varying emotional states
- Making conscious food choices
- Developing an awareness of hunger and satiety cues
- Cultivating self-acceptance [93]

Interviews with women who participated in such programs revealed a transformation from emotional and behavioural extremes, disembodiment and self-loathing to the cultivation of greater self-awareness, acceptance and self-compassion [94].

2.2.5.2 Chronic Illness

Mindfulness has been found to improve mood, anxiety and coping and prognostic markers in people dealing with major and life-threatening or debilitating illnesses such as various types of cancer [95, 96] and multiple sclerosis [97, 98].

Although depression has been found to be a poor prognostic factor for people with chronic illness such as breast cancer [99], it has yet to be demonstrated that mindfulness by itself, which improves depression, prolongs survival. There are, however, some promising findings pointing in that direction. For example, women with breast cancer who have MBSR training re-established healthy immune and cytokine production levels (it had an anti-inflammatory effect) and reduce cortisol levels – all good prognostic signs. This was associated with improved quality of life and increased coping effectiveness [80]. Even more interesting is the effect on telomeres (see below). Short telomeres are a poor prognostic sign for breast cancer, and telomere length in the mindfulness intervention group was maintained over time, whereas it decreased for control group [100].

Combining the health benefits of meditation with the direct health benefits of facilitating healthy lifestyle change may be a winning combination. Dean Ornish and his team demonstrated that a meditation-based lifestyle program was associated with the reversal of cardiovascular disease (CVD). The Ornish program [101] was the first demonstration ever that, given the right conditions, CVD is a reversible illness as the program improved quality of life as well as producing better clinical outcomes [102]. People with already established CVD were divided into two groups. The control group had routine medical care only. The intervention group had the routine medical care plus the Ornish lifestyle program consisting of:

- Group support
- Stress management including meditation and yoga
- A low-fat vegetarian diet
- Moderate exercise
- Stopping smoking

Most patients with conventional care alone slowly deteriorated over the 12 months, but the intervention group improved – they reversed their CVD as shown via an angiograph and their symptoms decreased. Improvement was directly related to the amount of lifestyle change in a dose-response manner. The average cost savings were $58,000 per patient because patients who went through the program were less likely to be admitted to hospital, have heart attacks, require bypass surgery or use more medications [103]. Enhancing mental health and coping with stress better were contributors to good CVD outcomes. Since poor mental health and high stress contribute to returning to an unhealthy lifestyle, this program nipped those problems in the bud [104]. A 5-year follow-up of Ornish program patients showed that the divergence between the two groups widened [105].

In a further ground-breaking series of studies, Ornish and his team studied men with early prostate cancer who chose to watch and wait while being monitored rather than have cancer treatments they may not have been needed. The men who chose to watch and wait were randomised into either a 'lifestyle' (experimental) group or a 'usual treatment' (control) group who were not encouraged to make lifestyle changes [106]. At the 2-year follow-up, 27 % (13/49) of patients in the control group went on to require cancer treatment because of disease progression. Only 5 % (2/43) of patients in the lifestyle group went on to require cancer treatment because of disease progression. Most of the lifestyle group, in fact, had reversal of a range of cancer markers, including PSA (prostate-specific antigen) [107]. Again, the improvements were consistent with a dose-response, meaning the greater the lifestyle change, the greater the improvements. They also measured prostate cancer gene expression and found that it was down-regulated by lifestyle change [108]. Comprehensive lifestyle change also increased telomerase activity compared to the men who just stayed on their usual lifestyle [109]. A 5-year follow-up on this same group of men has looked at the long-term effects of lifestyle change on telomere length. The intervention group have increased their telomere length, whereas it had decreased in the control group – this is the genetic equivalent of reversing the ageing process. Previous to this study, it was not known to be possible to regrow telomeres. The more the men adhered to healthy lifestyle, the longer their telomere was [110].

2.2.5.3 Lifestyle Change

Facilitating healthy lifestyle change is a prerequisite for the prevention and management of nearly all the chronic illness which are so common with ageing and Westernised lifestyle. Doing this better through mindfulness suggests an indirect means whereby these practices may have a positive effect on physical health.

Research on the effectiveness of suppression approach versus a mindfulness approach for smoking cessation found that the mindfulness group reduced smoking and had a far more stable mood, whereas the group trying to suppress the urge to smoke found that their moods significantly declined [111]. Suppressing an urge tends to draw more attention to it, whereas observing it with less reactivity has the opposite effect. This is sometimes called 'urge surfing'. A subsequent study on the effect of mindfulness meditation training versus relaxation training among smokers found that 2 weeks of meditation training produced a 60% reduction in smoking, but there was no reduction in the relaxation control group. Resting-state brain scans showed increased activity for the meditation group in the anterior cingulate (associated with attention) and prefrontal cortex, brain areas related to self-control [112].

Mindfulness/acceptance-based psychotherapy has been found to be helpful for relapse prevention in alcohol and other forms of substance abuse in part because common triggers for relapse, such as negative mood, distress and craving, are reduced [113–115]. Vipassana meditation, also called insight meditation, has been studied for addiction among prison inmates, which led to a decrease in alcohol-related problems and psychiatric symptoms and increases in positive psychosocial outcomes [116].

2.2.5.4 Chronic Pain

Mindfulness-based programs for people living with chronic pain have demonstrated a significant reduction in pain, fatigue and insomnia and improved function, mood and general health for people with chronic pain syndromes [117–119]. Hypervigilance and emotional reactivity are associated with a significant increase in pain; therefore, the main explanation for mindfulness being beneficial is the reduced emotional reactivity which has the effect of reducing the fixation on painful stimuli and the suffering associated with it [120, 121].

2.2.5.5 Mindfulness and Immune Functioning

Mindfulness has been found to alter the regulation of inflammatory pathways on an epigenetic level which may represent the mechanisms underlying the therapeutic potential of mindfulness-based interventions for the treatment of chronic inflammatory conditions [122]. Meditation down-regulates genes associated with inflammation and enhances the activity of genes associated with healthy immunity, i.e. healthy regulation of the immune system [123]. Mindfulness and compassion meditation practices are also associated with reduced inflammation [124] and may therefore be important in the management of a wide range of inflammatory and autoimmune illnesses like asthma, arthritis, dermatitis, multiple sclerosis and inflammatory bowel disease. Other examples relevant to cancer have already been provided.

A trial evaluating the effects of mindfulness meditation on the incidence, duration and severity of acute respiratory infections (ARI) found that the number and severity of ARIs was significantly reduced and the number of days off work related to ARIs was reduced by over 75 % [125].

2.3 Genetics

One relatively new and exciting field of research relates to the impact of the mind and mindfulness training on genetics. This is another example of epigenetics – the factors that influence how genes express themselves.

A little like the plastic bits on the end of shoelaces, telomeres are caps on the end of chromosomes that keep them from unravelling. They naturally shorten with age and are an indicator of biological age and the risk of illnesses associated with ageing like cancer, heart disease and dementia. In 2004, it was first noted in a study on healthy premenopausal women that prolonged psychological stress was associated with 9–17 years of additional ageing as measured by telomere length [126] which has major implications for how, at the cellular level, stress may promote earlier onset of age-related diseases. Since that time, a whole range of factors have been found to shorten telomere length more rapidly including work stress, pessimism, poor sleep and internalising racial discrimination and, importantly in the context of mindfulness, a wandering mind [127].

Mindfulness meditation has been shown to slow genetic ageing and enhance genetic repair as measured by the stimulation of telomerase (the enzyme that repairs telomeres) [128–130]. This has major implications for the future risk of chronic illness. Activation of the relaxation response through a variety of meditative techniques has been found to produce changes in the expression of genes associated with the activation of the stress response as well [131].

2.4 Conclusion

Taken altogether, mindfulness can be seen as high-level clinical skill, a therapeutic intervention, an aid to education and as a tool for improved educational outcomes and self-development. As such, there is a good case for it being a core part of clinician training. Effective mindfulness programs need to not only focus on individuals but also on the environments and systems within which health practitioners work and patients are helped.

References

1. Epstein RM. Mindful practice. JAMA. 1999;282(9):833–9.
2. Epstein R, Siegel D, Silberman J. Self-monitoring in clinical practice: a challenge for medical educators. J Cont Educ Health Prof. 2008;28(1):5–13.
3. Epstein RM. Mindful practice in action (II): cultivating habits of mind. Fam Syst Health. 2003;21:11–7.
4. Sibinga EM, Wu AW. Clinician mindfulness and patient safety. JAMA. 2010;304(22):2532–3.
5. Thammasitboon S, Thammasitboon S, Singhal G. Diagnosing diagnostic error. Curr Probl Pediatr Adolesc Health Care. 2013;43(9):227–31. doi:10.1016/j.cppeds.2013.07.002.
6. Hallowell EM. Overloaded circuits: why smart people underperform. Harv Bus Rev. 2005;83(1):54–62, 116.
7. McEvoy SP, Stevenson MR, Woodward M. The contribution of passengers versus mobile phone use to motor vehicle crashes resulting in hospital attendance by the driver. Accid Anal Prev. 2007;39(6):1170–6.
8. Tossell CC, Kortum P, Shepard C, Rahmati A, Zhong L. You can lead a horse to water but you cannot make him learn: smartphone use in higher education. Br J Educ Tech. 2015;46(4):713–24. doi:10.1111/bjet.12176.
9. Stothart C, Mitchum A, Yehnert C. The attentional cost of receiving a cell phone notification. J Exp Psychol Hum Percept Perform. 2015;41(4):893–7. doi:10.1037/xhp0000100.
10. Lutz A, Brefczynski-Lewis J, Johnstone T, Davidson RJ. Regulation of the neural circuitry of emotion by compassion meditation: effects of meditative expertise. PLoS One. 2008;3(3):e1897. doi:10.1371/journal.pone.0001897.
11. Lutz A, Greischar LL, Perlman DM, Davidson RJ. BOLD signal in insula is differentially related to cardiac function during compassion meditation in experts vs. novices. Neuroimage. 2009;47(3):1038–46. doi:10.1016/j.neuroimage.2009.04.081.
12. Lee TM, Leung MK, Hou WK, Tang JCY, Yin J, So K-F, et al. Distinct neural activity associated with focused-attention meditation and loving-kindness meditation. PLoS One. 2012;7(8):e40054. doi:10.1371/journal.pone.0040054.
13. Beckman HB, Wendland M, Mooney C, Krasner MS, Quill TE, Suchman AL, et al. The impact of a program in mindful communication on primary care physicians. Acad Med. 2012;87(6):815–9. doi:10.1097/ACM.0b013e318253d3b2.
14. Beach MC, Roter D, Korthuis PT, Epstein RM, Sharp V, Ratanawongsa N, et al. A multicentre study of physician mindfulness and health care quality. Ann Fam Med. 2013;11(5):421–8. doi:10.1370/afm.1507.

15. Dobkin PL, Bernardi NF, Bagnis CI. Enhancing clinician well-being and patient-centred care through mindfulness. J Contin Ed Health Profs. 2015 (in press).
16. Dobkin PL, editor. Mindful medical practice: clinical narratives and therapeutic insights. Switzerland: Springer International Publishing; 2015.
17. Willcock SM, Daly MG, Tennant CC, Allard BJ. Burnout and psychiatric morbidity in new medical graduates. Med J Aust. 2004;181(7):357–60.
18. Cooke GPE, Doust JA, Steele MC. A survey of resilience, burnout, and tolerance of uncertainty in Australian general practice registrars. BMC Med Educ. 2013;13:2. doi: 10.1186/1472-6920-13-2.
19. Epstein RM, Krasner MS. Physician resilience: what it means, why it matters, and how to promote it. Acad Med. 2013;88(3):301–3. doi:10.1097/ACM.0b013e318280cff0.
20. Dyrbye LN, Massie Jr FS, Eacker A, Harper W, Power D, Durning SJ, et al. Relationship between burnout and professional conduct and attitudes among US medical students. JAMA. 2010;304(11):1173–80. doi:10.1001/jama.2010.1318.
21. Fahrenkopf AM, Sectish TC, Barger LK, Sharek PJ, Lewin D, Chiang VW, et al. Rates of medication errors among depressed and burnt out residents: prospective cohort study. BMJ. 2008;336(7642):488–91. doi:10.1136/bmj.39469.763218.BE.
22. Regehr C, Glancy D, Pitts A, Leblanc VR. Interventions to reduce the consequences of stress in physicians: a review and meta-analysis. J Nerv Ment Dis. 2014;202(5):353–9. doi:10.1097/NMD.0000000000000130.
23. West CP, Dyrbye LN, Rabatin JT, Call TG, Davidson JH, Multari A, et al. Intervention to promote physician well-being, job satisfaction, and professionalism: a randomized clinical trial. JAMA Intern Med. 2014;174(4):527–33. doi:10.1001/jamainternmed.2013.14387.
24. Krasner MS, Epstein RM, Beckman H, Suchman AL, Chapman B, Mooney CJ, et al. Association of an educational program in mindful communication with burnout, empathy, and attitudes among primary care physicians. JAMA. 2009;302(12):1284–93. doi:10.1001/jama.2009.1384.
25. Asuero AM, Queraltó JM, Pujol-Ribera E, Berenguera A, Rodriguez-Blanco T, Epstein RM. Effectiveness of a mindfulness education program in primary health care professionals: a pragmatic controlled trial. J Cont Educ Health Prof. 2014;34(1):4–12. doi:10.1002/chp.21211.
26. Irving JA, Park-Saltzman J, Fitzpatrick M, Dobkin PL, Chen, Affiliated with Department of Counselling Psychology, McGill University A, Hutchinson T. Experiences of health care professionals enrolled in mindfulness-based medical practice: a grounded theory model. Mindfulness. 2014;5:60–71.
27. Garneau K, Hutchinson T, Zhao Q, Dobkin PL. Cultivating person-centered medicine in future physicians. Eur J Pers-Centred Healthc. 2013;1(2):468–77.
28. Breines JG, Chen S. Self-compassion increases self-improvement motivation. Pers Soc Psychol Bull. 2012;38(9):1133–43. doi:10.1177/0146167212445599. Epub 2012 May 29.
29. Crane C, Crane RS, Eames C, Fennella MJV, Silvertonb S, Williams JMG, et al. The effects of amount of home meditation practice in mindfulness based cognitive therapy on hazard of relapse to depression in the staying well after depression trial. Behav Res Ther. 2014;63:17–24. doi:10.1016/j.brat.2014.08.015.
30. Phang CK, Mukhtar F, Ibrahim N, Keng SL, Mohd Sidik S. Effects of a brief mindfulness-based intervention program for stress management among medical students: the Mindful-Gym randomized controlled study. Adv Health Sci Educ Theory Pract. 2015;20(5):1115–34. doi:10.1007/s10459-015-9591-3. Epub 2015 Feb 20.
31. Monshat K, Khong B, Hassed C, Vella-Brodrick D, Norrish J, Burns J, et al. A conscious control over life and my emotions: mindfulness practice and healthy young people. A qualitative study. J Adolesc Health. 2013;52(5):572–7. doi:10.1016/j.jadohealth.2012.09.008.
32. Taren AA, Gianaros PJ, Greco CM, Lindsay EK, Fairgrieve A, Brown KW, et al. Mindfulness meditation training alters stress-related amygdala resting state functional connectivity: a randomized controlled trial. Soc Cogn Affect Neurosci. 2015;10(12):1758–68. doi:10.1093/scan/nsv066. Epub 2015 Jun 5.

33. Reiner K, Granot M, Soffer E, Lipsitz JD. A brief mindfulness meditation training increases pain threshold and accelerates modulation of response to tonic pain in an experimental study. Pain Med. 2015. doi:10.1111/pme.12883.

34. Mrazek MD, Franklin MS, Phillips DT, Baird B, Schooler JW. Mindfulness training improves working memory capacity and GRE performance while reducing mind wandering. Psychol Sci. 2013;24(5):776–81. doi:10.1177/0956797612459659.

35. Ramsburg JT, Youmans RJ. Meditation in the higher-education classroom: meditation training improves student knowledge retention during lectures. Mindfulness. 2014;5(4): 431–41.

36. Hassed C, de Lisle S, Sullivan G, Pier C. Enhancing the health of medical students: outcomes of an integrated mindfulness and lifestyle program. Adv Health Sci Educ Theory Pract. 2009;14:387–8.

37. Slonim J, Kienhuis M, Di Benedetto M, Reece J. The relationships among self-care, dispositional mindfulness, and psychological distress in medical students. Med Educ Online. 2015;20:27924. doi:10.3402/meo.v20.27924.

38. Warnecke E, Quinn S, Ogden K, Towle N, Nelson MR. A randomised controlled trial of the effects of mindfulness practice on medical student stress levels. Med Educ. 2011;45(4):381–8. doi:10.1111/j.1365-2923.2010.03877.x.

39. McKenzie SP, Hassed CS, Gear JL. Medical and psychology students' knowledge of and attitudes towards mindfulness as a clinical intervention. Explore (NY). 2012;8(6):360–7. doi: 10.1016/j.explore.2012.08.003.

40. Zenner C, Herrnleben-Kurz S, Walach H. Mindfulness-based interventions in schools-a systematic review and meta-analysis. Front Psychol. 2014;5:603. doi:10.3389/fpsyg.2014.00603.

41. Ashcraft MH, Kirk EP. The relationships among working memory, math anxiety, and performance. J Exp Psychol Gen. 2001;130(2):224–37.

42. Beilock SL, Carr TH. When high-powered people fail: working memory and "choking under pressure". Math Psychol Sci. 2005;16(2):101–5.

43. Morrison AB, Goolsarran M, Rogers SL, Jha AP. Taming a wandering attention: short-form mindfulness training in student cohorts. Front Hum Neurosci. 2014;7:897. doi:10.3389/fnhum.2013.00897.

44. Greenberg J, Reiner K, Meiran N. "Mind the trap": mindfulness practice reduces cognitive rigidity. PLoS One. 2012;7(5):e36206. Epub 2012 May 15.

45. Opie J, Chambers R, Hassed C, Clarke D. Data on Monash 2013 medical students' personality, mindfulness, study engagement and wellbeing. 2015 (In preparation).

46. Bellinger DB, DeCaro MS, Ralston PA. Mindfulness, anxiety, and high-stakes mathematics performance in the laboratory and classroom. Conscious Cogn. 2015;37:123–32. doi:10.1016/j.concog.2015.09.001.

47. Dobkin PL, Laliberté V. Being a mindful clinical teacher: can mindfulness enhance education in a clinical setting? Med Teacher. 2014;36(4):347–52.

48. Flook L, Goldberg SB, Pinger L, Bonus K, Davidson RJ. Mindfulness for teachers: a pilot study to assess effects on stress, burnout, and teaching efficacy. Mind Brain Educ. 2013; 7(3):182–95.

49. Siegel D. The mindful brain: reflection and attunement in the cultivation of well-being. New York: WW Norton; 2007.

50. Doige N. The brain that changes itself: stories of personal triumph from the frontiers of brain science. New York: Viking Penguin; 2007.

51. Kornfield J, Siegel D. Mindfulness and the Brain: a professional training in the science and practice of meditative awareness. Sounds True Inc Audio Learning Course. 2010.

52. Kilpatrick LA, Suyenobu BY, Smith SR, Bueller JA, Goodman T, Creswell JD, et al. Impact of mindfulness-based stress reduction training on intrinsic brain connectivity. Neuroimage. 2011;56(1):290–8. doi:10.1016/j.neuroimage.2011.02.034.

53. Tang YY, Hölzel BK, Posner MI. The neuroscience of mindfulness meditation. Nat Rev Neurosci. 2015;16(4):213–25. doi:10.1038/nrn3916.

54. Hölzel BK, Carmody J, Evans KC, et al. Stress reduction correlates with structural changes in the amygdala. Soc Cogn Affect Neurosci. 2010;5(1):11–7.
55. Zeidan F, Johnson SK, Diamond BJ, David Z, Goolkasian P. Mindfulness meditation improves cognition: evidence of brief mental training. Conscious Cogn. 2010;19(2):597–605. epub 2010 Apr 3.
56. Hölzel BK, Carmody J, Vangel M, Congleton C, Yerramsetti SM, Gard T, et al. Mindfulness practice leads to increases in regional brain gray matter density. Psychiatry Res. 2011; 191(1):36–43.
57. Pagnoni G, Cekic M. Age effects on gray matter volume and attentional performance in Zen meditation. Neurobiol Aging. 2007;28(10):1623–7.
58. Lazar SW, Kerr CE, Wasserman RH, Gray JR, Greve DN, Treadway MT, et al. Meditation experience is associated with increased cortical thickness. Neuroreport. 2005;16(17): 1893–7.
59. Landau SM, Marks SM, Mormino EC, Rabinovici GD, Oh H, O'Neil JP, et al. Association of lifetime cognitive engagement and low β-amyloid deposition. Arch Neurol. 2012;69(5): 623–9.
60. Scarmeas N, Levy G, Tang MX, Manly J, Stern Y. Influence of leisure activity on the incidence of Alzheimer's disease. Neurology. 2001;57(12):2236–42.
61. Friedland RP, Fritsch T, Smyth KA, Koss E, Lerner AJ, Chenet CH, et al. Patients with Alzheimer's disease have reduced activities in midlife compared with healthy control-group members. Proc Natl Acad Sci U S A. 2001;98(6):3440–5.
62. McEwen BS. Protection and damage from acute and chronic stress: allostasis and allostatic overload and relevance to the pathophysiology of psychiatric disorders. Ann N Y Acad Sci. 2004;1032:1–7.
63. Park ER, Traeger L, Vranceanu AM, Scult M, Lerner JA, Benson H, et al. The development of a patient-centered program based on the relaxation response: the Relaxation Response Resiliency Program (3RP). Psychosomatics. 2013;54(2):165–74. doi:10.1016/j.psym. 2012.09.001.
64. Whittle S, Allen NB, Lubman DI, Yücel M. The neurobiological basis of temperament: towards a better understanding of psychopathology. Neurosci Biobehav Rev. 2006;30 (4):511–25.
65. Whittle S, Yap MB, Yücel M, Fornito A, Simmons JG, Barrett A, et al. Prefrontal and amygdala volumes are related to adolescents' affective behaviors during parent-adolescent interactions. Proc Natl Acad Sci U S A. 2008;105(9):3652–7. doi:10.1073/pnas.0709815105.
66. Whittle S, Yücel M, Fornito A, Barrett A, Wood SJ, Lubman DI, et al. Neuroanatomical correlates of temperament in early adolescents. J Am Acad Child Adolesc Psy. 2008; 47(6):682–93. doi:10.1097/CHI.0b013e31816bffca.
67. Visser TA, Ohan JL, Whittle S, Yücel M, Simmons JG, Allen NB. Sex differences in structural brain asymmetry predict overt aggression in early adolescents. Soc Cogn Affect Neurosci. 2014;9(4):553–60. doi:10.1093/scan/nst013. Epub 2013 Feb 27.
68. Farb NA, Anderson AK, Segal ZV. The mindful brain and emotion regulation in mood disorders. Can J Psychiatry. 2012;57(2):70–7.
69. Witkiewitz K, Lustyk MK, Bowen S. Retraining the addicted brain: a review of hypothesized neurobiological mechanisms of mindfulness-based relapse prevention. Psychol Addict Behav. 2013;27(2):351–65. doi:10.1037/a0029258.
70. Tang YY, Posner MI. Tools of the trade: theory and method in mindfulness neuroscience. Soc Cogn Affect Neurosci. 2013;8(1):118–20. doi:10.1093/scan/nss112.
71. Chiesa A, Serretti A. A systematic review of neurobiological and clinical features of mindfulness meditations. Psychol Med. 2010;40(8):1239–52. doi:10.1017/S0033291709991747.
72. Hamilton JP, Farmer M, Fogelman P, Gotlib IH. Depressive rumination, the default-mode network, and the dark matter of clinical neuroscience. Biol Psychiatry. 2015;78(4):224–30. doi:10.1016/j.biopsych.2015.02.020.
73. Simic G, Babic M, Borovecki F, Hof PR. Early failure of the default-mode network and the pathogenesis of Alzheimer's disease. CNS Neurosci Ther. 2014. doi:10.1111/cns.12260.

74. Brewer JA, Worhunsky PD, Gray JR, Tangc Y-Y, Weberd J, Kobera H. Meditation experience is associated with differences in default mode network activity and connectivity. Proc Natl Acad Sci U S A. 2011;108(50):20254–9.
75. Taylor VA, Daneault V, Grant J, Scavone G, Breton E, Roffe-Vidal S, et al. Impact of meditation training on the default mode network during a restful state. Soc Cogn Affect Neurosci. 2013;8(1):4–14. doi:10.1093/scan/nsr087.
76. Goyal M, Singh S, Sibinga EM, Gould NF, Rowland-Seymour A, Sharma R, et al. Meditation programs for psychological stress and well-being: a systematic review and meta-analysis. JAMA Intern Med. 2014;174(3):357–68. doi:10.1001/jamainternmed.2013.13018.
77. Ma SH, Teasdale JD. Mindfulness-based cognitive therapy for depression: replication and exploration of differential relapse prevention effects. J Cons Clin Psychol. 2004;72(1):31–40.
78. Teasdale JD, Moore RG, Hayhurst H, Pope M, Williams S, Segal ZV. Metacognitive awareness and prevention of relapse in depression: empirical evidence. J Cons Clin Psychol. 2002;70(2):275–87.
79. Rubia K. The neurobiology of meditation and its clinical effectiveness in psychiatric disorders. Biol Psychol. 2009;82:1–11.
80. Witek-Janusek L, Albuquerque K, Chroniak KR, Chroniak C, Durazo-Arvizu R, Mathews HL. Effect of mindfulness based stress reduction on immune function, quality of life and coping in women newly diagnosed with early stage breast cancer. Brain Behav Immun. 2008;22:969–81.
81. Way BM, Creswell JD, Eisenberger NI, Lieberman MD. Dispositional mindfulness and depressive symptomatology: correlations with limbic and self-referential neural activity during rest. Emotion. 2010;10(1):12–24.
82. Biegel GM, Brown KW, Shapiro SL, Schubert CM. Mindfulness-based stress reduction for the treatment of adolescent psychiatric outpatients: a randomized clinical trial. J Cons Clin Psychol. 2009;77(5):855–66.
83. Cohen L, Warneke C, Fouladi RT, Rodriguez MA, Chaoul-Reich A. Psychological adjustment and sleep quality in a randomized trial of the effects of a Tibetan yoga intervention in patients with lymphoma. Cancer. 2004;100(10):2253–60.
84. Britton WB, Haynes PL, Fridel KW, Bootzin RR. Polysomnographic and subjective profiles of sleep continuity before and after mindfulness-based cognitive therapy in partially remitted depression. Psychosom Med. 2010;72(6):539–48.
85. Goldin PR, Gross JJ. Effects of mindfulness-based stress reduction (MBSR) on emotion regulation in social anxiety disorder. Emotion. 2010;10(1):83–91.
86. Mayo-Wilson E, Dias S, Mavranezouli I, et al. Psychological and pharmacological interventions for social anxiety disorder in adults: a systematic review and network meta-analysis. Lancet Psychiatry. 2014;1(5):368–76. doi:10.1016/S2215-0366(14)70329-3.
87. Davis LW, Strasburger AM, Brown LF. Mindfulness: an intervention for anxiety in schizophrenia. J Psychosoc Nurs Ment Health Serv. 2007;45(11):23–9.
88. Chadwick P, Hughes S, Russell D, Russell I, Dagnan D. Mindfulness groups for distressing voices and paranoia: a replication and randomized feasibility trial. Behav Cogn Psychother. 2009;37(4):403–12. Epub 2009 Jun 23.
89. Dobkin PL, Irving JA, Amar S. For whom may participation in a Mindfulness-Based Stress Reduction program be contraindicated? Mindfulness. 2012;3(1):44–50.
90. Polusny MA, Erbes CR, Thuras P, et al. Mindfulness-based stress reduction for posttraumatic stress disorder among veterans: a randomized clinical trial. JAMA. 2015;314(5):456–65. doi:10.1001/jama.2015.8361.
91. Kimbrough E, Magyari T, Langenberg P, Chesney M, Berman B. Mindfulness intervention for child abuse survivors. J Clin Psychol. 2010;66(1):17–33. doi:10.1002/jclp.20624.
92. Kristeller J, Hallett C. An exploratory study of a meditation-based intervention for binge eating disorder. J Health Psychol. 1999;4:357–63.
93. Kristeller JL, Wolever RQ. Mindfulness-based eating awareness training for treating binge eating disorder: the conceptual foundation. Eat Disord. 2011;19(1):49–61.
94. Proulx K. Experiences of women with bulimia nervosa in a mindfulness-based eating disorder treatment group. Eat Disord. 2008;16(1):52–72.

95. Sharplin GR, Jones SB, Hancock B, Knott VE, Bowden JA, Whitford HS. Mindfulness-based cognitive therapy: an efficacious community-based group intervention for depression and anxiety in a sample of cancer patients. Med J Aust. 2010;193(5 Suppl):S79–82.
96. Matousek RH, Dobkin PL. Weathering storms: a cohort study of how participation in a Mindfulness-Based Stress Reduction program benefits women after breast cancer treatment. Current Oncol. 2010;17(4):62–70.
97. Grossman P, Kappos L, Gensicke H, D'Souza M, Mohr DC, Penner IK, et al. MS quality of life, depression, and fatigue improve after mindfulness training. A randomized trial. Neurology. 2010;75:1141–9.
98. Bogosian A, Chadwick P, Windgassen S. Distress improves after mindfulness training for progressive MS: a pilot randomised trial. Mult Scler. 2015;21(9):1184–94. Mar 12. pii: 1352458515576261.
99. Giese-Davis J, Collie K, Rancourt KMS, Neri E, Kraemer HC, Spiegel D. Decrease in depression symptoms is associated with longer survival in patients with metastatic breast cancer: a secondary analysis. J Clin Oncol. 2011;29(4):413–20.
100. Carlson LE, Beattie TL, Giese-Davis J, Faris P, Tamagawa R, Fick LJ, et al. Mindfulness-based cancer recovery and supportive-expressive therapy maintain telomere length relative to controls in distressed breast cancer survivors. J Alt Comp Med. 2014;20(5):A24–5. doi:10.1089/acm.2014.5060.abstract.
101. Ornish DD. Dean Ornish's program for reversing heart disease: the only system scientifically proven to reverse heart disease without drugs or surgery. New York: Random House; 1990.
102. Ornish D, Brown SE, Scherwitz LW, Billings JH, Armstrong WT, Ports TA, et al. Can life-style changes reverse coronary heart disease? Lancet. 1990;336:129–33.
103. News. US insurance company covers lifestyle therapy. BMJ. 1993;307(465). doi:10.1136/bmj.307.6902.463. http://www.bmj.com/content/bmj/307/6902/463.full.pdf.
104. Penninx BW, Beekman AT, Honig A, Deeg DJ, Schoevers RA, van Eijk JT, et al. Depression and cardiac mortality: results from a community-based longitudinal study. Arch Gen Psychiatry. 2001;58(3):221–7.
105. Ornish D, Scherwitz L, Billings J, Gould L, Merritt TA, Sparler S, et al. Intensive lifestyle changes for reversal of coronary heart disease. JAMA. 1998;280:2001–7.
106. Ornish D, Weidner G, Fair WR, Marlin R, Pettengill EB, Raisin CJ, et al. Intensive lifestyle changes may affect the progression of prostate cancer. J Urol. 2005;174(3):1065–9; discussion 1069–70.
107. Frattaroli J, Weidner G, Dnistrian AM, Kemp C, Daubenmier JJ, Marlin RO, et al. Clinical events in prostate cancer lifestyle trial: results from two years of follow-up. Urology. 2008;72(6):1319–23. doi:10.1016/j.urology.2008.04.050.
108. Ornish D, Magbanua MJ, Weidner G, Weinberg V, Kemp C, Green C, et al. Changes in prostate gene expression in men undergoing an intensive nutrition and lifestyle intervention. Proc Natl Acad Sci U S A. 2008;105(24):8369–74. doi:10.1073/pnas.0803080105.
109. Ornish D, Lin J, Daubenmier J, Weidner G, Epel E, Kemp C, et al. Increased telomerase activity and comprehensive lifestyle changes: a pilot study. Lancet Oncol. 2008;9(11):1048–57. doi:10.1016/S1470-2045(08)70234-1.
110. Ornish D, Lin J, Chan JM, Epel E, Kemp C, Weidner G et al. Effect of comprehensive lifestyle changes on telomerase activity and telomere length in men with biopsy-proven low-risk prostate cancer: 5-year follow-up of a descriptive pilot study. Lancet Oncol. 2013. doi:10.1016/S1470-2045(13)70366-8. pii: S1470-2045(13) 70366-8.
111. Rogojanski J, Vettese LC, Antony MM. Coping with cigarette cravings: comparison of suppression versus mindfulness-based strategies. Mindfulness. 2011;2(1):14–26. doi:10.1007/s12671-010-0038-x.
112. Tang YY, Tang R, Posner MI. Brief meditation training induces smoking reduction. Proc Natl Acad Sci U S A. 2013;110(34):13971–5. doi:10.1073/pnas.1311887110.
113. Vieten C, Astin JA, Buscemi R, Galloway GP. Development of an acceptance-based coping intervention for alcohol dependence relapse prevention. Subst Abus. 2010;31(2):108–16.

114. Brewer JA, Sinha R, Chen JA, Michalsen RN, Babuscio TA, Nich C, et al. Mindfulness training and stress reactivity in substance abuse: results from a randomized, controlled stage I pilot study. Subst Abus. 2009;30(4):306–17.
115. Bowen S, Chawla N, Collins SE, Witkiewitz K, Hsu S, Grow J, et al. Mindfulness-based relapse prevention for substance use disorders: a pilot efficacy trial. Subst Abus. 2009;30(4):295–305.
116. Bowen S, Witkiewitz K, Dillworth TM, Chawla N, Simpson TL, Ostafin BD, et al. Mindfulness meditation and substance use in an incarcerated population. Psychol Addict Behav. 2006;20(3):343–7.
117. Kabat-Zinn J, Lipworth L, Burney R. The clinical use of mindfulness meditation for the self-regulation of chronic pain. J Behav Med. 1985;8(2):163–90.
118. Singh BB, Berman BM, Hadhazy VA, Creamer P. A pilot study of cognitive behavioral therapy in fibromyalgia. Altern Ther Health Med. 1998;4(2):67–70.
119. Astin JA, Berman BM, Bausell B, Lee WL, Hochberg M, Forys KL. The efficacy of mindfulness meditation plus Qigong movement therapy in the treatment of fibromyalgia: a randomized controlled trial. J Rheumatol. 2003;30(10):2257–62.
120. Perlman DM, Salomons TV, Davidson RJ, Lutz A. Differential effects on pain intensity and unpleasantness of two meditation practices. Emotion. 2010;10(1):65–71.
121. Ursin H, Eriksen HR. Sensitization, subjective health complaints, and sustained arousal. Ann NY Acad Sci. 2001;933:119–29.
122. Kaliman P, Alvarez-López MJ, Cosín-Tomás M, Rosenkranz MA, Lutz A, Davidson RJ. Rapid changes in histone deacetylases and inflammatory gene expression in expert meditators. Psychoneuroendocrinology. 2014;40:96–107. doi:10.1016/j.psyneuen.2013.11.004.
123. Black DS, Cole SW, Irwin MR, Breen E, St Cyr NM, Nazarian N, et al. Yogic meditation reverses NF-κB and IRF-related transcriptome dynamics in leukocytes of family dementia caregivers in a randomized controlled trial. Psychoneuroendocrinology. 2013;38(3):348–55. doi:10.1016/j.psyneuen.2012.06.011.
124. Pace TW, Negi LT, Adame DD, Cole SP, Sivilli TI, Brown TD, et al. Effect of compassion meditation on neuroendocrine, innate immune and behavioral responses to psychosocial stress. Psychoneuroendocrinology. 2009;34(1):87–98.
125. Barrett B, Hayney MS, Muller D, Rakel D, Ward A, Obasi CN, et al. Meditation or exercise for preventing acute respiratory infection: a randomized controlled trial. Ann Fam Med. 2012;10:298–9.
126. Epel ES, Blackburn EH, Lin J, Dhabhar FS, Adler NE, Morrow JD, et al. Accelerated telomere shortening in response to life stress. Proc Natl Acad Sci U S A. 2004;101 (49):17312–5.
127. Epel ES, Puterman E, Lin J, Blackburn E, Lazaro A, Mendes WB. Wandering minds and aging cells. Clin Psychol Sci. 2012. doi:10.1177/2167702612460234.
128. Epel E, Daubenmier J, Moskowitz JT, Folkman S, Blackburn E. Can meditation slow rate of cellular aging? Cognitive stress, mindfulness, and telomeres. Ann N Y Acad Sci. 2009; 1172:34–53.
129. Lavretsky H, Epel ES, Siddarth P, Nazarian N, Cyr NS, Khalsa DS, Lin J, Blackburn E, Irwin MR. A pilot study of yogic meditation for family dementia caregivers with depressive symptoms: effects on mental health, cognition, and telomerase activity. Int J Geriatr Psychiatry. 2012. doi:10.1002/gps.3790.
130. Schutte NS, Malouff JM. A meta-analytic review of the effects of mindfulness meditation on telomerase activity. Psychoneuroendocrinology. 2014;42:45–8. doi:10.1016/j.psyneuen. 2013.12.017.
131. Dusek JA, Otu HH, Wohlhueter AL, Bhasin M, Zerbini LF, Joseph MG, et al. Genomic counter-stress changes induced by the relaxation response. PLoS One. 2008;3(7):e2576.

References

Chapter 3
Applied Mindfulness in Medicine

3.1 Introduction

Mindfulness is a generic skill that has many applications, many of which are of great relevance to medical training and practice. The previous chapters provided an overview of mindfulness and some of the relevant research. This chapter will provide a practical description of how the attributes associated with mindfulness can be applied in medicine. We will not focus primarily on the benefits of mindfulness for medical students but will explore those that are of direct clinical relevance to doctors.

3.2 Communication Skills

One of the first things students learn in medical school is how to communicate effectively. Communication is not merely an exchange of information but is also an exchange between whole persons (patient and clinician) including their thoughts (e.g. expectations) and affective reactions (e.g. anxiety, hope). This includes interprofessional interactions as well.

A number of factors can impair the quality and efficiency of communication in medical settings such as tiredness, distraction, multitasking, time pressure, stress and emotional states. Although being mindful can help with factors like these, it does not make a doctor immune to them. Nevertheless, being mindful means being self-aware enough to notice one's own inner state making it possible to take it into account during clinical interactions. So, for example, a doctor might experience fatigue in the latter stages of a long shift but being aware of the fatigue provides the opportunity to be more vigilant at a time when it is easy not to listen, to care or to make clinical errors. A doctor may be in a clinical interaction where emotions like anger arise, but, again, the ability to be self-aware provides the opportunity to self-monitor and

© Springer International Publishing Switzerland 2016
P.L. Dobkin, C.S. Hassed, *Mindful Medical Practitioners*,
DOI 10.1007/978-3-319-31066-4_3

regulate those emotions in a way that is less likely to prejudice the clinical interaction or bias the interpretation of clinical information.

Spending time with someone is not merely a matter of being physically together; it entails being mentally and emotionally engaged as well. Patients tend to pick up very quickly when a doctor is not really listening and will either shut down, withhold or give cursory answers. A doctor not really being present with the patient communicates disrespect or lack of care. Of course, when it comes the time to offer recommendations regarding management, if the doctor has not been listening to the patient, the patient is far less likely to listen attentively to the doctor or to adhere to that advice.

Default mode is a common impediment to clear and empathic communication. This is commonly experienced when the patient is speaking but the doctor is unconsciously distracted by internal thought processes. For example, a doctor thinking about what question to ask next makes it easy not to listen to the answer to the question that was just asked. The patient answers the doctor's question, but the doctor either doesn't hear the answer at all or only takes in a superficial understanding of what the patient has just said without awareness of any of the nuances of what they said, how they said it or even what they didn't say. Genuine communication requires being fully present to the self, the other person and the context during an exchange. We call this 'mindful congruence' [1]. Cues during consultations can be very fleeting, subtle and easily missed. There may only be one chance to pick them up. If the doctor jumps ahead, thinking about other patients waiting to be seen, he or she may not be responsive to the patient in the room at that moment.

Many thoughts arise in a doctor's mind while working with patients. A mindful doctor can sift through them and select those that are relevant. For instance, it may be useful to mentally flag a question to ask which has been prompted by the patient's responses but, having noted it, remain attentive to what the patient is actually saying. This is different from rehearsing it. Such relevant thoughts need to be distinguished from irrelevant ones such as 'How long until lunch?' or 'I hope I get out of work on time today'.

One problematic form that default mode takes is sometimes called 'reloading' or 'rehearsing' which is to be impatiently waiting while someone else is speaking all the while internally rehearsing what we are going to say next. Thus, one misses what the other person is saying now; when two people are both reloading not much is heard or retained. This phenomenon is common during arguments.

To summarise, some of the key practical points in communicating mindfully include:

- Consciously pausing, no matter how briefly, between one clinical interaction and the next one
- Listening with an open, curious, quiet and attentive mind
- Noticing the 'how' not just the 'what' regarding communication by being attentive to body language and emotional states
- Creating an atmosphere of openness, emotional safety and non-judgment
- Refraining from reloading or rehearsing while a patient or colleague is speaking
- Ignoring passing thoughts that are not directly relevant to the current situation

- Understanding the difference between a tangential and a meaningful distraction
- Being comfortable with silence and knowing when to wait and not interrupt
- Creating a safe space for a person to speak naturally and authentically
- Question and exploring in a dialectic way that enables a patient to develop insight
- Knowing when and how to end a dialogue

Because meditation helps one become more aware of internal thought processes and where the attention is, the ability to communicate in a mindful way will be enhanced by the regular practice of mindfulness meditation.

3.3   Developing Empathy, Compassion and Self-Compassion

Being empathic and compassionate are key attributes in doctors that are valued highly by patients and their families. Yet it tends to be poorly taught in medical school and is either ignored or, if taught, it is done so in a formulaic way where the doctor has rehearsed phrases and behaviours but is not necessarily present and responsive to the other person's cues or existent needs.

Maintaining empathy and compassion in medicine is not easy; in fact, it is frequently undermined in the clinical environments that students and junior doctors are exposed to. Some clinicians may not see it as important. As modern medicine became more of a science, and pharmaceutical and technologically based care took centre stage, the 'soft' or more human aspects of care and compassion could be seen as secondary or the responsibility of someone other than the doctor. Then there are the competing demands of workplace stress (e.g. night shifts, heavy caseloads), the depersonalisation associated with of burnout, time pressures and self-preservation from vicarious stress to be overcome. To counteract erosion of empathy, mindfulness that incorporates self-compassion and its impact of relationships is becoming recognised as an important part of training.

The term vicarious stress or trauma is associated with the cost of caring for others and is the emotional residue of exposure that professionals have from working with people who have experienced significant trauma, pain, fear and terror [2]. It occurs when empathy arises but the practitioner becomes identified with the suffering of the other. For health practitioners this can predispose to carer or compassion fatigue and burnout particularly in fields of medicine such as oncology and intensive care where suffering and death are commonplace. One effect of vicarious stress is that the amygdala becomes activated which can impair decision-making and empathy. Unhelpful ways of dealing with vicarious stress include 'protecting' oneself by cutting off and becoming 'clinical' in a cold, removed or dissociated way. This is not the same as the non-attachment associated with being mindful. The other way of dealing with vicarious stress is to become overwhelmed, burned out and unable to continue in the job. Both are common in medicine but these two alternatives are not the only possible ways of dealing with vicarious stress.

As reviewed in Chap. 2, mindfulness has been associated with an increased empathic response but reduced activation of amygdala. In the formal practice of mindfulness meditation, we learn to sit initially with our own physical and emotional pain when it arises, but in a compassionate, equanimous, non-judgmental and non-reactive way while remaining aware of and open to its presence. Learning to be with and accept suffering within us makes it easier to witness and be open to other's suffering with a similar compassionate attitude. Recognising the inevitability of suffering and death does imply that we should remain passive or refrain from doing what may assuage suffering or save a life – if that is possible – rather, it means accepting the basic laws of nature and existence.

Being compassionate does not take more time. It can be shown in the simplest ways such as really meeting a person's eyes, the gentle touch of the hand, the nod that comes with really hearing what a person has said or just taking the moment to sincerely ask a person how they are and actually listening to their response. Such moments can be brushed off as not essential, but they are often the most important moments to patients and their families and can enrich and humanise the working life of a doctor enormously.

For a medical course to espouse the importance of compassion, but for a lack of compassion to be modelled in the academic and clinical environments into which students are enculturated, is to teach hypocrisy in medicine, not compassion. This issue, i.e. the culture of medicine, will be covered in Chap. 8.

3.4 Patient Satisfaction

Patients and their families recognise and respond to the more mindful patterns of communication and compassion. Patient satisfaction is a natural consequence of being truly present during the encounter. The motivation of the mindful doctor is not so much an anxiety about receiving patient approval. Furthermore, medicolegal problems are less likely to occur when the relationship between clinician and patient is healthy and respectful.

3.5 Clinical Skills in Motivation, Lifestyle and Stress Management

Nearly all of the major burdens of disease in developed countries, and increasingly in developing countries, are lifestyle and mental health related. Clinicians need to know how to educate patients about the importance of healthy lifestyles and how to make necessary changes (e.g. diet and exercise in diabetes) for the prevention or management of chronic illness.

A number of the elements of mindfulness are easily learned and can be applied in clinical situations. For example, communication has already been discussed. The core elements of motivational interviewing like being patient-centred, questioning, being non-judgmental, eliciting insight and resolving ambivalence are all entirely complementary to a mindful consultation style. Such aptitudes are best learned by observing them modelled by experienced tutors and clinicians [3] rather than hearing or reading about them in class or texts.

Not every clinician considers himself or herself a mental health professional, but every clinician should, by being interested and attentive, be able to recognise the presence of stress-related illnesses or mental health problems, raise the potential for mindfulness and how it might be relevant for the patient, explain the principles of mindfulness-based therapeutic approaches and know where to refer the patient for mindfulness training when appropriate.

An increasing number of clinicians are becoming proficient in teaching meditation practices to patients, but, from a therapeutic perspective, it is essential for a doctor to have significant training (discussed in Chap. 7) and personal experience in mindfulness if it is going to be used in more challenging therapeutic settings like major depression and anxiety, chronic pain or coping with debilitating or life-threatening illness. Knowing when to refer to more experienced and skilled practitioners, and knowing which clinical situations mindfulness might be contraindicated [4], is important lest it do harm by being poorly delivered.

3.6   Clinical Reasoning, Decision-Making and Prevention of Errors

Fatigue, emotional states like anxiety and anger, cognitive bias, haste, multitasking and distraction are common causes of poor clinical decisions and clinical and diagnostic errors. Among other things, fatigue reduces vigilance and cognitive processing; stress and amygdala activation can narrow situational awareness and hijack cognitive centres; cognitive bias unconsciously distorts perception of incoming data; and haste, multitasking and distraction can lead to premature conclusions being reached and relevant information being missed.

Mindfulness can counter these problems in a number of ways. Firstly, self-awareness is a prerequisite for self-monitoring, being able to recognise and take mental states like fatigue or stress into account and thus being able to allow for them. It protects against the automatic pilot state where errors are made but not noticed, or at least not until an unfortunate outcome may have occurred. The ability to observe the presence of one's inner state may not make it go away, but it does allow for the doctor to be able to make allowance for it, self-correct or choose more discerningly how to express oneself.

Similarly, when cognitive biases such as confirmation, anchoring or sunk-cost bias arise, they remain unconscious but influential if we are operating on automatic pilot. Being mindful implies being aware of cognitive processes as they arise which affords the ability to not take any unconscious thought or assumption as a fact. As a result, it makes it possible not to be so influenced by them or to act on them prematurely. So, for example, a family medicine practitioner may be seeing a number of young children being brought in with low-grade fevers in the middle of winter, and when another comes in, the clinician may quickly jump to a conclusion that it is another child with a cold. This then colours how the clinician interprets the clinical signs. A more mindful practitioner would observe the assumption as it occurs and not take it as a fact, although it may be relevant as a probability diagnosis. He or she is more likely to be able to actually see what signs are present in the ears and throat and to listen attentively to the lungs when the stethoscope is applied rather than to just see and hear what he or she expects to see and hear.

One of the problems associated with time pressures and haste is the unconscious desire for quick and oftentimes premature closure of diagnoses and management decisions. Clearly, there is a difference between decisions that need to be made quickly such as in emergency situations, and those that are being made in haste because the clinician is uncomfortable with clinical uncertainty or because they feel oppressed by work pressures. The former can be done mindfully in response to the context; the latter can be unmindful and unnecessary and can result in maladaptive reactions to context.

Other simple strategies can also be such as taking a few moments to notice the physical and emotional state when about to walk into an examining room, not multitasking and being able to steady oneself when feeling hurried and hassled.

3.7 Efficiency, Time Management and Sustainable Performance

Efficiency is a combination of the amount of energy, time or resources it takes to complete a task versus the outcome. A lack of mindfulness tends to lead to poor use of energy, time and resources. For example, we can expend far more energy in procrastination, anticipation and worry about a task than it actually takes to complete the task. This can be circumvented by engaging with the actual task rather than ruminating about it. We can waste time by making errors, having to reread things or repeat questions because the mind continually wanders off. This can be sidestepped by aiming and sustaining attention while the task is being completed. Thus, one engages with the task fully using only the energy and time necessary to complete it.

The effect of distraction and multitasking can be precarious in complex environments such as hospitals. There is the constant bombardment with stimuli like beepers and phones, work flows that are frequently disrupted, and there is an oftentimes emotionally charged environment to navigate.

Some tips for practically integrating mindfulness to enhance efficiency include:

- Moving quickly when one needs to, but not being mentally hurried as one does so. Being mentally hurried is generally a result of getting ahead of the present moment rather than just moving through a complex task moment by moment and step by step.
- Refraining from complex multitasking even when the temptation is great.

- Efficiently switching attention when the need arises. This is not multitasking. Efficient attention switching is necessary in fast-moving and complex situations such as emergencies of performing complex medical procedures particularly in teams. Attention remains agile but focused on one thing at a time, and not distracted by irrelevant environmental cues.
- Being less affected by distracter influence. At any given moment, there are a few elements in the environment that are relevant and many that are irrelevant. To be uninfluenced and uninterested by what is not relevant is what we do when we are in the 'zone' or 'flow state'.
- When possible, take control over the environment. Can stimuli be reduced? Simplify the environment.
- Performing complex tasks like writing a medical report or assignment, reading an article or taking a complex history is far easier when the flow of that activity is not being constantly interrupted by questions, phone calls or emails. If possible, perform complex tasks without interruption and compartmentalise time by moving on to those other activities like returning phone calls and emails or responding to questions after the complex task has been completed. If the interruption is necessary, such as in emergencies, then do the best one can to gently, not reactively, shift to the new task and then come back to the previous one when the opportunity arises.

3.8   Workplace Stress and Burnout

As seen in Chaps. 1 and 2, the medical profession tends to have poorer mental health than the general population, in part as a result of the characteristics of the people selected to enter the profession, and in part because of the demands that go with the job itself. There are a number of mindfulness-based strategies that can help to reduce workplace stress and the risk of burnout among doctors. These are also relevant for medical students coping with study pressures.

Stress, anxiety and depression are perpetuated when the mind is allowed to drift into default mode of worry and rumination. For example, one can increase workplace pressure enormously in anticipating the multitude of things one might have to do before the end of the day rather than just engaging with the one thing in front of us at any given moment. Worry about work misuses the energy required to do the job mostly through nervous tension and leaves one much more depleted at the end of the day. Conserve energy by moving through the day one step, one job, one moment at a time. By all means, make a list of the jobs that need attending to if necessary, but attend to those jobs one at a time. Conserve energy. When walking down the corridor, opening a door, writing a letter or driving the car, use the minimum of energy required to do it.

It also helps to have a very brief moment of mindfulness meditation between the completion of one job and the commencement of another. Depending on time and place, this can be anything from a few seconds to a minute or two, for example, to take a few moments to notice where the attention is, what is the state of mind and body, before stepping up to deal with a medical emergency. Take a minute to punctuate the day after completing the notes for the last patient in an outpatient session and before heading up to the ward to review inpatients.

It is imperative to patiently and gently keep orientating the attention, through the senses, back to the present moment. This should be done in an accepting and self-compassionate way, like training a puppy with a consistent but loving manner.

Working mindfully includes recognising times when we need to have a break. When having a break at work or when at home after work, avoid the temptation to keep filling each moment of the day with worry about work. That having been said, there is a need to discern between those things that are coming to mind because they need attention and those that are merely worry, rumination or distraction. If something is coming to mind because it needs attention, now, then to orientate attention back to reading the book or watching the television is not necessarily mindfulness. It may be avoidance. Avoidance will not lead to a release of tension and a quietening of the mind – quite the opposite. What will lead to a release of tension and a quieter mind is to attend to the job that is being avoided.

Worry often captures attention because it masquerades as something useful, like planning and preparation. One can mindfully plan for the future just as one can mindfully reflect on the past. One may intentionally, consciously and purposefully prepare for some upcoming event or job. That may be useful and necessary, but that is different to the mental churning after the necessary preparation has taken place. In worry, one is mentally living events before they have happened and being distracted from the priorities of the moment. Similarly, reflecting objectively and purposefully on past experience in order to gain insight is different from the rumination so often associated with burden and regret. Such rumination often obscures the lesson rather than reveals it.

Aim to conserve energy. 'Right effort', i.e. just enough, is key for energy management. It is important to recognise when it's time to take a break. Allow this to include real spaces in the day (e.g. turning off all devices and eating mindfully) and not giving into the temptation to fill each moment of the day with something to do. In other words, allow time for being rather than doing constantly in order to recharge [5].

Long hours and shift work are demanding aspects of medical practice. Many find it hard to switch off at the end of a long day or an overnight shift. Sitting down to stop is one thing, but if the mind is racing, this does not allow for rest. Taking some time for mindfulness meditation helps transition between work and home, and home and work. However, should one be unsettled after a demanding day's work, it can be challenging to concentrate. Then, it may be more useful to take a mindful walk or practice yoga.

Of course, if after making changes one still finds that work is leading to burnout or having a negative effect on mental health, then one needs to ask the question whether medicine is the right profession, or the area of medicine one is engaged in is the right fit for one's talents and motivation. 'Sunk-cost bias' can influence one's decision to continue a direction in life that may not be serving one well. Being able to let go of the attachment to the job and what one has previously invested in it, and to be authentic to the needs and direction of life that is truly calling us, is a very mindful thing to do.

3.9 Inter-professional Relationships and Teamwork

Inter-professional relationships can be one of the most fulfilling or most stressful parts of a career in medicine. A few important and practical aspects of how to do this mindfully are, first, when a colleague is speaking, listen and don't multitask. If you really do need to complete an important task, then do it first and then have the conversation. It is better to do that than have a half-engaged conversation and interrupt the flow of an important job.

Second, learn to be more self-aware and less reactive in your interactions with colleagues. It is easy for unconscious or reactive anger to escalate workplace conflict rather than resolve it. If we are mindful, then we are likely to have a deeper insight into why colleagues may be acting in the way they are. For example, somebody's impatience with us may be a result of them having just had an unpleasant experience which we are unaware of. It doesn't excuse rudeness, but it at least helps us to be more forgiving and tolerant.

Third, we need to be aware of how we relate and respond to others and choose to do that in such a way that supports rather than undermines them. That mindfulness assists us in developing self-respect, and self-compassion makes sense only if that translates into how we treat others, and not just medical colleagues, but respect for all people working across different levels of the hospital or clinical environment including allied health professionals, administrative staff and those working in service sectors. Rather than becoming part of the problem by perpetuating a dysfunctional workplace culture of disrespect, bullying or abuse, it is possible to be part of the solution.

3.10 Work Engagement

The opposite of work engagement is sometimes called 'presenteeism' – being physically present but mentally absent when at work. That is close to a definition of what it means to be unmindful.

Mindfulness is associated with greater work and study engagement [6]. Things that enhance work engagement include contextual features such as timely, supportive and accurate feedback, meaningful tasks, positive relationships with colleagues, task autonomy and opportunities to use skills fully [7]. Contextual features that detract from work engagement include excessive workload, work-home conflicts and emotional and physical demands that exceed the person's perceived ability to meet them. The key features that mindfulness offers is the ability to be less affected by work stressors that impair work engagement, a greater ability to focus and be present when at work, an ability to be absorbed in the work as it is happening and the ability to leave it mentally when it is time to.

3.11   Finding Meaning in Work

Finding meaning in one's work is closely associated with satisfaction with life in general and being able to positively cope with the negative aspects of work life. Merely working for secondary gains like financial rewards or status does not sustain one particularly in times of adversity. Conversely, doing something that is intrinsically meaningful and important for its own sake can help to put the ups and downs of working life in a larger perspective and minimise their impact. To be mindful means to be more in touch with our intrinsic motivation and being able to act in a way more authentic to core values.

References

1. Hutchinson TA, Dobkin PL. Discover mindful congruence. Le Spécialiste. 2015;17(1):31–2.
2. American Counseling Association. Vicarious trauma [Internet]. Fact Sheet #9 [cited 2015 Nov 6]. Available from: http://www.counseling.org/docs/trauma-disaster/fact-sheet-9---vicarious-trauma.pdf.
3. Dobkin PL, Laliberté V. Being a mindful clinical teacher: can mindfulness enhance education in a clinical setting? Med Teach. 2014;36(4):347–52.
4. Dobkin PL, Irving JA, Amar S. For whom may participation in a mindfulness-based stress reduction program be contraindicated? Mindfulness. 2012;3(1):44–50.
5. Epstein RM. Just being. West J Med. 2001;174(1):63–5.
6. Atkins PWB, Hassed C, Fogliati VJ. Mindfulness improves work engagement, wellbeing and performance in a university setting. In: Burke RJ, Page KM, Cooper CL, editors. Flourishing in life, work and careers. Individual wellbeing and career experiences. Cheltenham: Edward Elgar Publishing Limited; 2015. p. 193–209. Chapter 10.
7. Christian MS, Garza AS, Slaughter JE. Work engagement: a qualitative review and test of its relations with task and contextual performance. Pers Psychol. 2011;64(1):89–136. doi:10.1111/j.1744-6570.2010.01203.x.

Chapter 4
How Mindfulness Has Been Integrated into Three Medical School Curriculums

4.1 Introduction

As mentioned in Chap. 1, medical schools have been introducing mindfulness to their students in various ways – from single lectures, to workshops and electives, to complete courses. Very few have been able to integrate it into their core curriculum. This chapter features three prominent universities that have succeeded in doing this. The authors (from each university) describe not only *what* they teach but also the *evolution* of their respective programs. Naturally, the narratives differ as they each had to adapt to the norms and needs of their respective institutions. Rather than have these serve as templates, they are meant to show what is achievable when program developers are committed to this endeavour, are able to communicate the rationale to faculty and are able to creatively integrate mindfulness content within an already existing curriculum. These model programs illustrate that it took time and patience to integrate mindfulness into mainstream Western medical school classrooms and practicums.

The featured mindfulness programs described below are in chronological order of their being introduced into core medical curriculum. They are:

1. Monash University, Melbourne, Australia
2. The University of Rochester, Rochester, USA
3. McGill University, Montreal, Canada

Each one of these programs has had to be contextualised within a medical program; to be made relevant to local circumstances, interests and needs; and to reflect the nature of the person/people who developed it. Some of this is intentional, some of it is accidental and some is opportunistic in the sense that the advocate for mindfulness in the curriculum seizes the opportunities they have within the parts of the medical curriculum over which they have some influence.

Like a multifaceted diamond, each program reflects different applications of mindfulness and aspects of what it means to be a mindful medical practitioner.

© Springer International Publishing Switzerland 2016
P.L. Dobkin, C.S. Hassed, *Mindful Medical Practitioners*,
DOI 10.1007/978-3-319-31066-4_4

At Monash University, for example, appearing early on in the medical course as it does, there is a significant emphasis on self-care and managing stress and lifestyle issues. It is founded on a holistic philosophy of health care and does extend in a limited way in later years into Mindful Medical Practice. In the Rochester program, appearing later in the medical course, the importance of self-care is recognised, but there is a far greater emphasis placed on how mindfulness creates a mindful medical practitioner. As such, it is the foundation for high-level clinical skills and decision-making. These two programs were developed independently. The McGill program was developed later. It was able to draw on the experience from other medical schools like Monash and Rochester, but gave its program its own local flavour. At McGill there is more overt emphasis on where it sits within whole person care and the doctor-patient relationship and its application for Mindful Medical Practice.

What these three programs illustrate is the importance of being *faithful to the philosophy* of mindfulness but *flexible in the form* of how it is communicated and delivered. Sometimes these two things – faithfulness and flexibility – are confused by those wishing to teach mindfulness, i.e. by being too flexible with the philosophy and too faithful to the form. This is a mistake on both counts. For example, those who have limited experience and don't understand mindfulness deeply enough can be loose or imprecise with the underlying philosophy. This impacts what they are teaching and how they are teaching it. They may be presenting what they think is mindfulness, or be conflating it with things that are not consistent with mindfulness, and mislead the student as a result. There is the potential that mindfulness teaching and practice will lose its way. Equally, one could be too faithful to the form. For example, 'A mindfulness course has to start with a particular exercise on week 1, students have to practice meditation for 40 minutes a day, the course has to include mindful yoga etc'. All these things are useful, but may not meet the students where they are, be seen as clearly relevant to their professional training or suit the amount of curriculum time available. Inflexibility is not faithfulness; it is rigidity, and rigidity potentially interferes with creativity and the ability to adapt mindfulness teaching to the local needs, opportunities and context [1]. For example, just taking a standard MBSR course and expecting to introduce it into a medical curriculum may not be a good fit and may bring resistance from students or faculty. This is not a negative reflection on the value of MBSR or to suggest that MBSR principles should not be followed, but merely a suggestion to work with, not against, the prevailing environment. From that initial engagement, mindfulness teaching may evolve and expand over time.

4.2   Monash University: Craig Hassed

Monash University in Melbourne, Australia, has a large medical school with a 5-year undergraduate medical degree and well over 500 medical students in each year level. Mindfulness has been integrated into the Monash University core under-graduate medical curriculum since 1991. It was probably the first medical school in the world to do this. Initially, the content was limited and focused on a one-off 2-h workshop on meditation-based stress management in the first year of the course. At this time, there was also a 12-week mindfulness and mind-body medicine elective that students could choose if they wished to extend their interest in this field. This elective proved to be one of the most popular offered to students.

The profile of mindfulness was already popular with the students because it was meeting significant needs, like being able to manage the stress associated with their studies, so when a new medical curriculum was being developed in 2000 the opportunity arose to develop a more significant and integrated student well-being program. Taking the first opportunity, this program was to be embedded into the first year of the course as a part of the Personal and Professional Development theme. The subsequent mindfulness-based lifestyle unit was called the Health Enhancement Program (HEP) and was delivered for the first time in 2002.

The HEP begins in the second half of the first semester of the first year and is framed around the ESSENCE acronym with ESSENCE standing for:

- *Education* – not just medical education but being more educated about ourselves, our motivations and health behaviours
- *Stress management* – the mindfulness component of the HEP including the principles of mind-body medicine
- *Spirituality* – exploring where we find meaning and purpose in life whether through religion, relationships, work, philanthropy or other ways
- *Exercise* – the importance of physical activity for mental and physical health and healthy ageing
- *Nutrition* – the importance of healthy nutrition for mental and physical health and healthy ageing
- *Connectedness* – the importance of social support, healthy relationships and a sense of community
- *Environment* – the importance of a healthy physical, educational and social environment

The students learn about the ESSENCE model [2] and how it applies in health care by first applying it to themselves before they consider how it can be applied to patients. The model is framed in terms of the ESSENCE of health, the ESSENCE of self-care as well as the ESSENCE of preventing or managing chronic illness. The students can't truly understand how important these issues are for their patients if they can't appreciate how important they are for themselves. The objectives of the HEP are to foster behaviours, attitudes, skills and knowledge conducive to:

- Learning personal self-care strategies for managing stress and maintaining a healthy lifestyle
- Understanding and applying mindfulness-based strategies for personal and professional use
- Enhancing student's physical health
- Laying the foundations for future clinical skills in stress and lifestyle management
- Integrating HEP content with biomedical, psychological and social sciences

- Understanding the mind-body relationship
- Developing a holistic approach to health care
- Developing peer support among the student body
- Enhancing academic and future clinical performance
- Improving communication skills

In the HEP, there are nine lectures providing an overview of the HEP covering its relevance, the evidence base and clinical importance of mind-body medicine, behaviour change strategies and mindfulness-based therapies, framed around the various elements of the ESSENCE acronym. This evidence base is very important because if the students are not acquainted with the science and applications of such topics that are not normally included in medical curricula, then they will tend to marginalise them in their minds and think of this as a 'soft' part of the medical curriculum.

The lectures, based on the science, rationale and theory, are then supported by six 2-h tutorials in groups of 15–16 students each. Theory without practice is like a lecture on hydration without drinking the water – it is not actually satisfying or transformative. The lectures are important as they are the way of 'getting the horse to the water', but the tutorials are where the students 'drink the water' and can begin to reflect on the impact on their lives.

The tutorial content each week includes 1 h on the Mindfulness-Based Stress Release Program (SRP) [3] and 1 h dedicated successively to each of the other elements of the ESSENCE model. The SRP had been successfully implemented in postgraduate training courses through the Royal Australian College of General Practitioners since 1991 and had been used for distance learning through the Monash University Diploma of Family Medicine since 1993. It has also been used in the early 2000s as an elective program at Harvard Medical School [4].

The SRP incorporates:

1. *Brief formal mindfulness meditation practices*: Mindfulness, having been introduced in the lecture, is then taken up practically in the tutorials. Students explore what it means to be mindful and what is the cost of unmindfulness (i.e. distraction, disengagement and inattention) in their lives. Arising from this is the rationale as to why being mindful may be useful in life. They are then invited to participate in a mindfulness 'experiment' – a brief guided meditation practice – by the tutor. They then reflect on, and learn from, their experience, whatever it may be. Between tutorials, students are encouraged to take up the formal practice of mindfulness meditation beginning with 5 min twice a day, preferably before and after their university day. They are then encouraged to increase it to 10 min twice daily if they feel motivated to do so. These practices for a few minutes are called 'full stops' to punctuate their day, but they are also encouraged to practice numerous 'commas' throughout their day of 15–60 s particularly as they transition from one activity to another.
2. *The informal practice of being mindful in daily life*: There is little point in being mindful for 10 min a day during meditation practice and then being unmindful for the remaining 23 h and 50 min. So the students are encouraged to apply mindfulness informally by observing where their attention is as they go about

their daily life, whether studying, conversing, eating, walking or anything else. They are invited to notice what comes with being mindful or unmindful. It includes noticing what is taking place when they are stressed, procrastinating or engaged in leisure activities. Being mindful is taken in a very broad sense. It is not just about concentrating when they are doing something like studying, but includes foci such as self-awareness, noticing their internal mental state and default mode, what is taking place in their bodies during the day, what it feels like to be on automatic pilot and the presence or lack of empathy while interacting with others.

3. *A series of four cognitive practices*: These are aimed at raising awareness of the mental processes underpinning stress, emotional states such as anger and depression and what underpins poor performance. The 'big four' cognitive topics we explore are:

   • Perception – being able to mindfully distinguish between imagination and present moment 'reality'
   • Letting go (non-attachment) – the ability to observe thoughts, feelings, sensations, events and possessions without attachment to them
   • Acceptance – the attitude with which we meet our internal and external experiences, including the impact of self-criticism or self-compassion
   • Presence of mind – learning to be in the present moment and coming out of the recreated past or imagined future

4. *In-class mindfulness experiments*: These 'experiments' are to enhance students' inquiry into mindfulness and to help integrate it with other elements of the ESSENCE model and curriculum more broadly. They include experiences such as a mindful communication exercise, mindful eating and exercising mindfully. There are experiments on the impact of multitasking and how to deal with distractor influence. Students also participate in a series of role-plays where they need to take 'patients' through the lifestyle change strategies they are applying to themselves and to communicate the basic principles of mindfulness to someone. These latter exercises are linked to what they will be expected to be able to do in upcoming OSCE exam stations.

Weekly 'homework' or practice is given in the form of personally applying the mindfulness strategies in daily life. The following week, the group explores their experiences and insights. Class discussion is driven by the questions, issues and insights of the students, not the tutor. They give it the context by taking the generic principles and practices of mindfulness and applying them in particular ways that are meaningful to them. The tutoring style is very much a Socratic, eliciting one consistent with the principles of mindful inquiry and motivational interviewing. Students are not expected to accept or reject mindfulness content or principles, but they are encouraged to test them. The level of personal application remains entirely the choice of individual student, but personal experience is seen as the most effective way to achieve deep learning, integration, self-awareness and personal benefit. Core knowledge and a basic understanding of mindfulness principles are expected, but personal practice mindfulness and healthy lifestyle change, while encouraged, are not coerced. Privacy is respected and students are never asked to say or write anything that they are not comfortable to share in tutorials or journals. The approach to self-care and building clinical skills is pragmatic, and over the weeks, the group members become increasingly open and supportive of each other. If students identify themselves to the tutor as having significant mental health, behavioural, academic or drug problems, this is treated confidentially, and they are referred to the appropriate faculty or student counselling or medical services because the program is not designed to be therapeutic for major health issues.

Support materials include an online student manual, the course text – The ESSENCE of Health – online readings including journal articles and guided meditation practices.

Throughout the HEP, students also maintain a weekly journal reflecting on their personal experiences, questions and insights of applying the course to themselves. The students write approximately 300 words on each of the mindfulness and lifestyle issues of the week. Journals are handed in to the tutor who returns them the following week with feedback and encouragement.

The journal is formative assessment and a hurdle requirement. It needs to be satisfactorily completed in order to pass the semester. The journal does not contribute a mark towards summative assessment because that would encourage students to write model answers to the reflective topics rather than honest, authentic ones. A student would be applauded, for example, if they authentically described their ambivalence or difficulty in practising mindfulness rather than giving a manufactured response in order to appear to be a model student.

Although the great majority of students report finding the HEP enjoyable and relevant, some find it philosophically challenging and not what they expected from a traditional course in biomedicine. Care is taken to deliver the program in such a way that it is seen as integral to clinical medicine rather than peripheral to it. Strategies to enhance this are:

- Provide an evidence-based lecture series.
- Core knowledge is integrated into weekly case-based learning to demonstrate clinical applications.
- Help students appreciate that mindfulness is important for being able to study effectively as well as to be an effective practitioner.
- Demonstrate how mindfulness is a skill underpinning effective decision-making, preventing cognitive bias and enhancing communication and prevention of errors.
- Make the content assessable with written (MCQs) and oral (OSCE) summative assessment integrated with other components of the medical course and formative (hurdle requirement) assessment related to the journal.

Mindfulness principles and skills are revisited and reinforced in later years of the curriculum when students are learning about enhancing clinical performance, improving communication skills and managing mental health problems. So, for example, mindfulness is emphasised as an important aspect of advanced communication skills in second year. It is revisited in the year third HEP which focuses on the mind-body and lifestyle management of chronic illness. It also arises in the general practice management of stress and psychiatric issues like mild to moderate depression and anxiety, or substance abuse in year 4.

Tutors are selected based on their personal commitment to the content as well as their professional experience in small-group teaching, behaviour change and mindfulness-based strategies. As described in Chap. 7, tutors are trained in how to deliver the HEP through having previous mindfulness training, participating in the HEP themselves and having a 3-h tutor briefing before the commencement of the HEP to orient them to the course structure and delivery.

Research on the Monash HEP suggests that over 90 % of students personally apply mindfulness in their own life. Although many students are inconsistent with their meditation practice, the majority enthusiastically take to the cognitive and informal practices. This is a very high uptake considering the students are not self-selected.

Research on the Monash HEP has found significant improvement in student mental health and quality of life even during high-stress periods of the semester like pre-exams [5]. All scales and subscales of the measures used (DASS, WHOQoL and the SCL-90) moved in a positive direction despite the fact that pre-course measures were in a low-stress period of semester and post-course measures were immediately prior to mid-year exams. A more recent study of students across the 5 years of the Monash medical course confirmed that dispositional mindfulness was associated with greater well-being and better self-care [6]. We have also found that the mindfulness component improves the students' study engagement right across the whole curriculum in the medical course [7]. Subsequently, Monash medical students have been found to be highly likely to recommend mindfulness to patients as adjunctive management for a wide variety of medical and mental health conditions when compared to medical students who do not have mindfulness content in their curriculum [8].

The ensuing level of interest in mindfulness more widely at Monash University has been such that in recent years other faculties have been motivated to include it into core curriculum. These faculties include Physiotherapy, Nursing, Dietetics, Occupational Therapy, Psychology, Pharmacy, Law, Information Technology, MBA, Business and Economics, and Education. Across the university, there are generic mindfulness programs open to all staff, an introduction to mindfulness for all new academic heads, weekly drop-in sessions on all campuses and online and open mindfulness courses and resources offered for Monash staff through the CEED (Continuing Educational Excellence Development) Framework and Internationally through FutureLearn [9]. For Monash students, outside of content within curriculum, there are also free Mindfulness for Academic Success (MAS) programs running year-round. Those who are interested to glimpse what is offered can view Mindfulness at Monash [10] or read Mindful Learning [11] where we describe the rationale and method of teaching mindfulness within educational settings.

4.3 University of Rochester School of Medicine and Dentistry: Michael Krasner

The mindfulness program at the University of Rochester School of Medicine and Dentistry is referred to as Mindful Practice. Developed in 2005–2007 and implemented in 2007–2008, Mindful Practice is a required mindfulness-based curriculum for all medical students during the third year of their education, the central year in which they are engaged in full-time clinical experiences. Its objectives are to address professional formation and enhance the student's capacity for building resilience and addressing burnout through a contemplative, reflective and self-care-oriented strategy. To our knowledge, it is the first required mindfulness curriculum in a US medical school.

As mentioned in the opening of this chapter, the conditions that shaped this curriculum and led to its placement in the undergraduate medical training program involved both faithfulness and flexibility. It occurred through circumstances and individuals coming together with a vision as well as a willingness (1) to engage the existing academic culture in a mindfulness-based approach to medical education and (2) to use the availability of a small amount of curricular time, with thoughtful consideration of the most skilful means to leverage those two.

4.3.1 Origins

This educational intervention was built on a strong biopsychosocial foundation already part of the educational culture at the University of Rochester School of Medicine and Dentistry. The biopsychosocial model was theorised by psychiatrist George L. Engel at the university and putatively discussed in a 1977 article where he posited 'the need for a new medical model' [12]. The biopsychosocial model was one of the first articulations affecting medical education that acknowledged what now there is little disagreement on the importance of understanding the effects of the workings of the body on the mind and of the effects of the workings of the mind on the body.

In 1999, Ronald Epstein, a faculty member in the Department of Family Medicine at the University of Rochester School of Medicine and Dentistry and a student of George Engel's biopsychosocial model, published an article entitled *Mindful Practice* [13]. In this article, Epstein defines Mindful Practice as *moment-to-moment purposeful attentiveness to one's own physical and mental processes during every day work with the goal of practising with clarity and compassion*. Mindful Practice refers to qualities of exemplary clinicians that transcend clinical specialty and clinical experience. These qualities include the ability to be present, attentive, and curious and to adopt a 'beginner's mind' and have the goal of greater awareness and insight into one's own work. Although Epstein argued that mindfulness can link relationship-centred care and evidence-based medicine and should be considered a characteristic of good clinical practice, other than recognising it in exemplary clinicians, there was no discussion for how to assist medical students to develop and cultivate these qualities.

Between 2000 and 2005, another faculty member, Michael Krasner from the Department of Medicine, had been teaching Mindfulness-Based Stress Reduction to several separate groups including patients, medical students and practising physicians. Several nearly simultaneous opportunities arose that brought Epstein, Krasner and a number of other faculty members together to consider ways to bring the qualities of Mindful Practice into the undergraduate, graduate and postgraduate medical educational experiences. This led to the creative efforts to develop the Mindful Practice program.

By 2004–2005 Epstein was involved in efforts at the Dean's office at the University of Rochester School of Medicine and Dentistry where he was engaged in the development of curricular materials to meet educational content imperatives put forth by the Liaison Committee on Medical Education (LCME) and the Accreditation Committee on Graduate Medical Education (ACGME). The LCME and ACGME are the authoritative accreditation bodies for medical schools and residency programs, respectively, in the United States, and among other content requirements that were declared was one that required medical schools and residency programs to address professionalism and professional formation. Epstein obtained funding to help develop these content areas from the Arthur Vining Davis Foundation, the Arnold Gold Foundation and the Mannix Foundation.

Meanwhile, Krasner led the team to obtain funding to develop a mindful communication program for practising physicians that addresses burnout and enhances well-being from the Physicians Foundation for Health Systems Excellence. With these resources combined, Epstein, Krasner and a team of faculty members from a variety of disciplines who had each participated in previous mindfulness-based training set about the task of designing, implementing and studying the resulting Mindful Practice program.

4.3.2 Components of the Mindful Practice Program

The overarching question facing this team as they developed the Mindful Practice program was how to design an intervention that can transform one's *way of being* as a physician or as a physician in training. That transformation very early on was perceived to include not only a change in how students relate to their patients but also to their colleagues and to themselves. Care and attention to oneself thus became a central tenet to becoming a better physician, and as a result to becoming more attentive and aware of the needs of patients.

The program can be conceptualised as Mindful Practice functioning as a container, with three *technologies* filling and supporting that container. These components, highly integrated one with the other, became the basis for the pedagogical approach. They include mindfulness meditation, narrative medicine and Appreciative

Inquiry. The Mindful Practice program is taught in 'modules' with each module focusing on a theme of relevance and challenge for the learners. Within each module, participants are invited to engage in mindfulness practices, the sharing of clinical narratives and the use of Appreciative Inquiry.

Mindfulness meditation is the medium through which narrative and appreciative dialogues operate. The quality of mindfulness, cultivated through the meditative practices, functions as an ever-present lens through which personal stories are contemplated, written, shared and discussed. The students are introduced to contemplative practices that cultivate mindfulness including the body scan, mindful movement, sitting meditation and walking meditation.

All of these formal practices are designed to enhance the participants' awareness of the stream of thoughts, the flow of feelings and the presence of sensations that are very often not noticed, yet inform action and behaviour from moment to moment. Through the enhancement of the awareness that develops from the regular practice of these mindfulness meditations, it becomes possible at times to step out of the *automatic pilot* mode of living and instead experience and act with greater awareness.

In order to assist the participants in applying the lessons learned through formal practice to their daily lives, participants are encouraged to bring the same quality of awareness to other activities, both in the classroom, during discussion, while developing and sharing narratives, when engaged in Appreciative Inquiry exercises, and also outside of the classroom, while engaged in life's activities, in particular in activities on their clinical clerkships. Supportive materials such as audio recordings of formal mindfulness meditation practices are provided to guide daily home exercises, and facilitators provide suggestions for awareness practices that can be accomplished easily, requiring only moments, while on the wards, in the classroom or at home.

Narrative medicine provides a way of understanding the personal connections between students and students' values and beliefs, how these become manifest in the physician-patient relationship and how that connection relates to the society in which it develops. According to Charon, narrative medicine helps imbue the facts and objects of health and illness with their consequences and meanings for individual patients and physicians [14].The use of narratives in medicine grants access to knowledge about the patient and about the practitioner himself/herself that would have otherwise remained out of reach. Narrative medicine in the Mindful Practice program includes the sharing of stories that arise from the students' clinical experiences and takes the form of reflection, dialogue and discussion in large and small groups, specific writing exercises, and journaling. Narratives are chosen by the students about their own personal experiences of caring for patients. Thus, the narratives are grounded in the real lived experiences of students, not in philosophical or rhetorical – what ifs.

Appreciative Inquiry (AI) strives to foster growth and change by focusing attention on existing capacities and prior successes in relationship building and problem solving (as opposed to an exclusive focus on problems and challenges). Much of medical training is problem-focused; patients are described in terms of problem lists, with little attention to recognising their strengths and resources. Students who witness poor clinical outcomes have little educational time spent exploring the presence of effective teamwork and joint decision-making present even in these experiences.

The theory behind AI is that identification, reinforcement and analysis of positive experiences with patients, families, working teams and with oneself are more likely to change behaviour in desired directions than the exclusive critique of negative experiences or failures [15]. Appreciative Inquiry involves the art and practice of asking unconditionally positive questions that strengthen the capacities to apprehend, anticipate and heighten positive potential. It is an inquiry tool that fosters imagination and innovation. The AI approach makes several assumptions: (1) for every person or group, there is something that is working; (2) looking for what works well and doing more of it is more motivating than looking for what doesn't work well and doing less of it; (3) what we focus on becomes our reality, and individuals and groups move towards what they focus on; (4) the language we use to describe reality helps to create that reality; (5) people have more confidence to journey to the future if they carry forward parts of the past; (6) we should carry forward the best parts of the past.

In the Mindful Practice curriculum, the first two steps of a traditional AI approach – *definition* and *discovery* – are integrated into the structure of interpersonal dialogues in the sharing of participants' narratives. Students learn to use AI techniques when engaged in appreciative dialogues, discussion and reflection of the narrative exercises. Thus, even though the themes of the modules are challenging ones, the students learn that within these experience lie relevant and accessible positive qualities that they possess, which can assist them in meeting future challenges and demands.

In addition to the integration of these three components – the cultivation of mindfulness through meditative practice, narratives related to clinically relevant themes and interpersonal dialogues influenced by Appreciative Inquiry – each module focuses on the participants developing a range of communication skills to enhance the capacity for storytelling and listening. The following themes form the basis of current modules in use in the Mindful Practice program:

- Noticing
- Responding to suffering
- Compassionate action
- When things go wrong
- Grief and loss
- Resilience
- The present moment
- Uncertainty
- Conflict
- Professionalism
- How doctors think
- Time
- Self-care and burnout
- Interpersonal mindfulness: awareness in action
- Finding balance at work and home
- Death and dying
- Teamwork and partnership

4.3.3 Faculty Development

It was recognised early in the developmental process that if this curriculum was to become a permanent and dynamic part of the medical student (and resident) experience, faculty from each of the clinical services in which the students are rotating should be facilitators. The reasoning may seem obvious, but it is worth mentioning. The qualities and skills promoted in the Mindful Practice curriculum for students to acquire should be important enough for faculty to acknowledge the same for themselves. Therefore, facilitators who embody these qualities through their own way of being as physicians and as teachers, and who represent these qualities and values as being core to their own clinical domains, can best represent this curriculum and teach it with the most relevance.

Over a year before the curriculum was rolled out into the third year clerkship experience, and given that there had already been a history of physician-focused Mindfulness-Based Stress Reduction programs that many academic and nonacademic physicians had attended, we identified faculty from the Departments of Medicine, Family Medicine, Neurology, Psychiatry and Surgery who might be interested in participating as facilitators. Several members from each of these departments agreed to participate in a year-long faculty development training program. This program included regular gatherings where this interdisciplinary group practised mindfulness meditation (all had at least taken an MBSR course previously or concurrently), with separate seminars on narrative medicine and Appreciative Inquiry. We are indebted to the participation of a number of colleagues who assisted in our faculty development process. They include the following:

- Michael Baime MD, Clinical Associate Professor of Medicine, University of Pennsylvania School of Medicine, Founder and Director of the Penn Program for Mindfulness.
- Clayton Baker MD, Clinical Associate Professor, Department of Medical Humanities and Bioethics, University of Rochester School of Medicine and Dentistry
- Rita Charon, MD, PhD, Executive Director, Program in Narrative Medicine, Professor of Clinical Medicine, Department of Medicine, College of Physicians and Surgeons of Columbia University
- Saki Santorelli EdD, MA, Executive Director, Center for Mindfulness, Director, Mindfulness-Based Stress Reduction Clinic, Professor of Medicine, Division of Preventive and Behavioural Medicine, University of Massachusetts Medical School
- Penny Williamson ScD, internationally recognised Facilitator, Educator and Coach for leaders and organisations in health care, founding Facilitator and Mentor for the national Center for Courage and Renewal and Associate Professor of Medicine, The Johns Hopkins University School of Medicine

The year-long training program also included practising teaching the modules to each other, with debriefing, critique and feedback given. After the year was completed, the program was rolled out live with the third year students and separately with residents. Drs. Epstein and Krasner personally observed each of the sessions, with specific feedback provided to the faculty involved. Additionally, the teaching faculty continued to meet regularly during the first year of the program for ongoing support, mindfulness practice and improvement of the modules.

4.3.4   Experience to Date

The Mindful Practice program at the University of Rochester School of Medicine and Dentistry for the third year medical students has been in place since 2008. Every medical student experiences a total of five 90-min sessions, beginning with an introductory session at the end of their second year during their comprehensive assessments and continuing throughout their third year clinical clerkships. Anecdotal experience suggests it to be a useful and relevant complement to the challenging clinical experiences of the third year, and it has been well accepted by faculty and medical school administration alike for its support of the LCME and ACGME requirements as well as its embodiment of the bio-psychosocial model, a part of the cultural fabric of the medical school.

Although specific outcomes relating to burnout, resilience and well-being have not been measured among medical students, the Mindful Practice program was studied among a group of primary care physicians in a year-long intensive, using the same curriculum, where outcomes of burnout, well-being and patient-centred qualities were measured. Published in JAMA in 2009, this program demonstrated sustained improvements in empathy, psychosocial orientation, burnout, mood and personality with increased emotional stability. These improvements appeared to be mediated by improvements in mindfulness [16]. Additionally, participants identified three areas that they felt accounted for the success of this intervention: it addressed professional isolation, it taught them useful skills (contemplative, narrative and appreciative skills), and it helped give themselves permission for self-care [17].

The Mindful Practice curriculum has been made available for interested individuals and institutions since its development, and for the past 6 years, the developers have offered residential retreat-like training programs for medical educators and other health professionals (see Chap. 7). Over 400 such individuals have attended from medical schools, universities and other health-care institutions on every continent. Components of Mindful Practice have influenced and have been integrated into over a dozen medical schools throughout the world.

4.3.5   Future Efforts

From the third year medical student perspective, although relevant to the skills necessary for healthy professional formation, the Mindful Practice curriculum represents a very minute portion of the educational experience during that formative year.

One of the challenges that we are beginning to address is to coordinate the sessions so that they occur in a sequential fashion, and over a relatively shorter period rather than being spread over the entire third year. Additional opportunities for students to engage in Mindful Practice on an elective and ongoing basis is being planned, as well as a rejuvenation of the faculty training through more unique faculty development activities, with recruitment of new Mindful Practice faculty.

Finally, educational outcomes related to professionalism, well-being, self-care, burnout and resilience should be included in future assessments of this program. These evaluations will help inform future module development and changes in timing and placement of the curriculum. We would like to see collaboration in collecting these and other outcomes data from the many institutions that have or are planning on implementing the Mindful Practice curriculum in their institutions.

For more information on this program, please visit www.mindfulpractice.urmc.edu.

4.4   The McGill Experience: Tom A. Hutchinson, Stephen Liben, and Mark Smilovitch

4.4.1   Origins

Our intent in teaching mindfulness began as a way of giving students skills and a way of being that would help them facilitate healing and the practice of whole person care. McGill Programs in Whole Person Care were established by Dr. Balfour Mount in 1999. Soon after it was set up, Drs. Mount and Kearney led a faculty working group on healing [18] that met over a 2-year period and came up with a proposal for teaching whole person care to McGill medical students. The proposal was accepted by the faculty who needed to respond to an accreditation report that identified deficiencies in the psychosocial aspects of the medical curriculum at McGill. The teaching of healing [19] was linked with the teaching of professionalism [20] in a physicianship curriculum [21]. From the onset, we were aware that mindfulness would be an important component of this teaching which led four of us to take a 1-week condensed MBSR course with Jon Kabat-Zinn and Sake Santorelli at the Center for Mindfulness in Worcester, followed by further courses with the same group. We began teaching what we had learned in Worcester combined with some content from the work of Virginia Satir on relationship [22] to faculty at McGill and health-care practitioners in Montreal [23] and in an elective 4-week course to fourth year medical students [24]. Overall, these initiatives were very well received and provided a base from which we began to introduce the teaching of mindfulness as a core component of the medical curriculum at McGill. We experienced some resistance in this process but were aided by the openness of the Dean and key members of the faculty. We were also aided by the creation of a new curriculum in 2013 that gave us the opening to teach an innovative course on Mindful Medical Practice to all medical students in the second year. Currently, we are teaching in all 4 years of the core curriculum at McGill.

4.4.2 When and What Do We Teach?

First Year From their first lecture on their first day in medical school, which focuses on professionalism and healing, and in five subsequent sessions in their first year, we clarify for students the difference between curing and healing [25] and give them examples and firsthand experiences of the healing process from both the patient's and the physician's perspective. This includes large class lectures, panel discussions with patients and physicians, films and small-group discussions. The aim is to make students familiar and open to healing as a central part of medical practice. It turns out this is not difficult because many of our students come with an openness, enthusiasm and longing to be part of this enlarged vision of medical practice. During the first year, we also introduce the concept of congruence and the need for any interaction with a patient to include the patient as a person, the physician as a person and the context [26]. In the last session of the first year when they review the difficulties in the year completed and the year to come, we introduce the idea of Mindful Medical Practice [13] as one concrete learnable way for them to be fully present with themselves, each other and in patient encounters. We preview at that point a course on Mindful Medical Practice (MMP) that we teach in the second year in the lead up to clerkship.

Second Year In second year, our primary teaching is a seven-consecutive-week MMP course [27] taught in groups of 20, 2 h per week. In this course, we teach mindfulness and congruent relating in a clinical context using brief didactic teaching, guided awareness exercises, narrative, role-plays, dyad interactions and large-group discussions. The topics of the individual session are:

1. Attention and Awareness: In this first session, we clarify intentions for the course and why a course on Mindful Medical Practice is relevant for their future careers. We then engage in exercises that demonstrate the learnable skill of managing distractions by honing attention and the polar opposites of multitasking and mindfulness.
2. Congruent Communication: We clarify the difference between reacting and responding and outline particular reactive stances that human beings unconsciously adopt in stressful interactions with another person. We clarify the relationship between mindfulness and congruent relating.
3. Awareness and Decision-Making: We explore three core concepts: (a) situational awareness and medical decision-making; (b) the role of emotion and cognition in decision-making; (c) mindful congruence as a learnable skill to prevent medical errors.
4. Clinical Congruence: We explore both cognitively and experientially through role-plays the core concepts of the following: features of the clinical context, the centrality of the diagnostic process to the structure of medical practice, the difference between healing and curing, clinical congruence and the role of mindfulness in clinical congruence.
5. Building Resilience: We clarify the concept of burnout and how some of the characteristics of medical professionals may lead to burnout. We explain the

'resilient zone' and its relationship to mindfulness. Using Insight Dialogue, we have students experience the power of active listening for the well-being of the person being listened to *and* to the person doing the listening.

6. Being with Suffering: In this class, we explore through cognitive discussion and experiential exercises the nature of suffering, helpful and unhelpful ways to be with suffering and the importance of death anxiety in our relationship to suffering. We have students experience how awareness of their own mortality can change their mindfulness.

7. Mindfully Congruent Practice in Clerkship and Beyond: In this final class, we explore the difference between knowing and actualizing. We clarify the importance of practice and commitment to self-care as a core aspect of medical practice. We use the iceberg metaphor as a way of helping students reflect on and share with each other their experience in the course and their thoughts and feelings with regard to their upcoming clinical clerkship.

The students are evaluated by attendance and participation, an essay describing their experience in the course and multiple-choice questions in the exam at the end of that section. We taught this course to all medical students at McGill for the first time in 2015. The vast majority of the essays were positive and insightful. The anonymous evaluations submitted by students had an overall score of 4.3/5.0. We will continue to teach this course and hope to use the base it provides to deepen the teaching that we are already doing in third and fourth years.

Third Year In third year, while students are heavily engaged in clinical activities during their clerkship, we teach several sessions. First, during a recall day, when students return from their individual clerkship rotations for whole-class teaching, we conduct panel discussions on the experience of the patient and the experience of the physician. In the first of these discussions, students hear about patients' best and worst experiences and what they have learned that they would like the students to know. In the second panel, which includes physicians at different stages in their careers, we ask physicians the same questions. There is considerable overlap and some differences between the sets of responses with the overriding message being the benefits and rewards to both patients and physicians of being present to the human relationship in medical care.

In a session focused on resilience in a clinical context [27] and conducted in 6 groups of 30 students at the simulation centre, we have each student experience a difficult interaction with a simulated supervisor or patient and then debrief the experience in both a small group (with two other students and a faculty tutor) and in a large group (all 30 students, 10 tutors and a facilitator). The aim of the session is to make them aware of their automatic reactions to a stressful interaction and by reflection to see ways they could change or modify their approach. The main framework for this instruction is the concept of mindful clinical congruence and the communication stances [26, 28]. We challenge students to stay mindful in these deliberately confronting situations. We have found these extremely intense sessions an excellent way to have students experience the value of mindfulness when the going gets tough in stressful clinical encounters. We are often amazed at what an effective job they do in staying mindful.

Fourth Year In this final year of medical school, we teach a 2 h session to the whole class as a summary of healing and professionalism and suggestions for how these should be brought into their transition to residency. With a changed curriculum in the process of implementation, a new transition to residency course will be introduced. We expect to use this opportunity to reinforce our teaching of mindfulness and its relevance to medical practice as our students make the transition to residency. As mentioned previously, an elective on Mindful Medical Practice is available to 20 students/year prior to graduation.

4.4.3   Our Aim in Teaching

In the Chico tapes [29], teacher and family therapist Virginia Satir says that the aim of all her teaching and instruction is to produce a sparkle in the eyes of the participants. We have very much the same aim. If that interest, enthusiasm and longing for something more can be touched, the rest follows easily. And we would say that our ability to elicit that response and sparkle in medical students at McGill has exceeded our expectations. Some examples include:

- Following a film on the life of psychiatric physician Viktor Frankl, students are deeply touched by Frankl's experience and end up forming a group to read and discuss his book 'Man's Search for Meaning'.
- In a discussion following the noticing red exercise in our first MMP class, a wild-eyed student recounts 'I was so focused on red that I would not have noticed how many of my colleagues were still in the room', an insight that we had not predicted but is highly relevant to clinical practice.
- A student reflects in one of the later MMP classes that she had known her colleagues in many contexts and knew, for instance, which beer they preferred but she had never gotten to know them *like this* – a developing sense of shared experience and community.
- In our simulation centre session, a student says that she sees her natural tendency is to please other people at the expense of her own well-being. She now realises that it is also at the expense of the other's well-being, and she sees an opening to change her response.

Are these random examples or do they have a common theme that has something to do with mindfulness and its relationship to medical practice? The common theme is getting students in touch with themselves, with their thoughts, feelings, expectations and most importantly their deep longings [30] that are in the final analysis what propelled them to medical school and will fuel their future careers. In our framework, the purpose of mindfulness is very simple – to put students deeply in touch with themselves and thereby foster their ability to relate deeply to themselves and to other people.

4.4.4 How Do We Teach?

We take this need to put students deeply in touch with themselves emotionally and experientially very seriously indeed. Whether or not the lecture, panel discussion, small-group session or other teaching format includes a specific reference to mindfulness, we are always, in how we conduct ourselves and relate to our students, attempting to inculcate this aspect of mindfulness into our teaching. We use an acronym partially inspired by the work of Heath and Heath [31] – surprise, engagement, emotional involvement and stories (SEES). Let us look at each of these in turn.

Surprise: Most students like most people in all contexts conduct their lives in a business-as-usual mode – what's for lunch, how long will this take, I should not have stayed up so late last night. Our first aim is to shock students out of this mode (it can be a mild shock) by introducing something unexpected. This can be anything from an unexpected video to start a class, an interactive exercise, skipping an opening meditation in favour of an interesting quote that we ask students to reflect on or a surprising piece of music. The key is to grab students' interest, and we find that the creativity in doing this is part of the joy of teaching and also puts a sparkle in our own eyes.

Engagement: This means that the students need to be working as hard as or harder than their teachers. We want to tap their energy by asking them questions (in large or small groups), getting them to interact in dyads, involving them in role-plays and engaging them in the give and take of disagreement and discussion. We have found that even in large groups, the whole group is more likely to be engaged when one or more of their peers is actively interacting in the teaching process. This is one of the reasons we sometimes use one of the students in the class as a member of discussion panels involving patients (there are always students who have been a patient) or physicians. It turns wisdom from on high to wisdom in which the students themselves have a stake and a contribution to make.

Emotional Involvement and Stories: We put these two together because we find that the best way to involve students emotionally is through stories, and stories provide the connection and coherence that tie a lecture or a small-group session together. We attempt to use stories that are authentic, are clinically relevant and have touched us in the same way we hope that they will touch our students. Some stories provide an overarching frame for a session, while others provide an illustration of a particular point that we wish to make. Interestingly, we find that stories that are fresh for us have more impact for students than stories we have repeated many times in the past and have become rote and stale. Students are presumably responding to our emotional involvement which shows in our facial expression, body language and other analogue communication, which cannot be faked [32].

4.4.5 A Safe Container

An aspect of teaching that we have found increasingly important is to create a safe space for students to experience mindfulness and its clinical relevance. There are two aspects to this, one that students initially welcome and the other less so. The more welcomed aspect concerns our attitude to students in the class. This is best described as an approach of Appreciative Inquiry [33]. We are always looking for what is valid and good about any comment or remark by a student and how this can be used to move the action forward for the whole class. We find that as students begin to trust this process, they open up, are more willing to risk and become more and more active participants.

There is a second aspect of safety that is less initially welcomed by students although we have found it absolutely essential for success. We approach our teaching with extreme seriousness and impose ground rules that set conditions for the students' participation in our small-group sessions: all classes start exactly on time; students are present and participating for the full duration of the class; all conversations, unless otherwise directed, are with the leader or facilitator; and strict confidentiality is observed for any personal revelations that students share in the class. Although some students initially resent these rules, we have found that they give our classes a momentum and effectiveness that would otherwise be lacking and provide the clarity and safety that we need to conduct these classes.

4.5 Conclusions

We teach mindfulness as a path to the facilitation of healing and whole person care for our students and the patients for whom they will provide care. This is an ongoing learning process in which our core teaching of mindfulness and healing has increased steadily over the past 15 years with wider and wider acceptance from faculty and students. We see this as an opportunity to change a whole new generation of doctors in a way that will help to fulfil our primary mission: *To transform western medicine by synergizing the power of modern biomedicine with the potential for healing of every person who seeks the help of a healthcare practitioner.* [34].

References

1. Dobkin PL, Hickman S, Monshat K. Holding the heart of MBSR: balancing fidelity and imagination when adapting MBSR. Mindfulness. 2014;5(6):710–8.
2. Hassed C. The essence of health: the seven pillars of wellbeing. Sydney: Random House; 2008.
3. Hassed C. Know thyself: the stress release program. Melbourne: Michelle Anderson Publishing; 2006.
4. Rosenthal JM, Okie S. White coat, mood indigo – depression in medical school. N Engl J Med. 2005;353(11):1085–8.
5. Hassed C, de Lisle S, Sullivan G, Pier C. Enhancing the health of medical students: outcomes of an integrated mindfulness and lifestyle program. Adv Health Sci Educ Theory Pract. 2009;14:387–98.

6. Slonim J, Kienhuis M, Di Benedetto M, Reece J. The relationships among self-care, dispositional mindfulness, and psychological distress in medical students. Med Educ Online. 2015;20:27924. doi:10.3402/meo.v20.27924.
7. Opie J, Chambers R, Hassed C, Clarke D. Data on Monash 2013 medical students' personality, mindfulness and wellbeing. 2015 (In preparation).
8. McKenzie SP, Hassed CS, Gear JL. Medical and psychology students' knowledge of and attitudes towards mindfulness as a clinical intervention. Explore (NY). 2012;8(6):360–7. doi:10.1016/j.explore.2012.08.003.
9. Mindfulness for Wellbeing and Peak Performance [Internet]. Australia; Monash University. 2015 [cited 8 Dec 2015]. Available from: https://www.futurelearn.com/courses/mindfulness-wellbeing-performance.
10. Mindfulness at Monash [Internet]. Australia; Monash University. 2012 [updated 10 Feb 2015; cited 8 Dec 2015]. Available from: https://monash.edu/counselling/mindfulness.html.
11. Hassed C, Chambers R. Mindful learning. Sydney: Exisle Publishing; 2014.
12. Engel GL. The need for a new medical model: a challenge for biomedicine. Science. 1977;196(4286):129–36.
13. Epstein RM. Mindful practice. JAMA. 1999;282(9):833–9. doi:10.1001/jama.282.9.833.
14. Charon R. Narrative medicine: honoring the stories of illness. New York: Oxford University Press; 2006.
15. Cooperider DL, Whitney D. Appreciative inquiry: a positive revolution in change. San Francisco: Berrett-Koehler Publishers; 2005.
16. Krasner MS, Epstein RM, Beckman H, Suchman AL, Chapman B, Mooney CJ, et al. Association of an educational program in mindful communication with burnout, empathy, and attitudes among primary care physicians. JAMA. 2009;302(12):1284–93. doi:10.1001/jama.2009.1384.
17. Beckman HB, Wendland M, Mooney C, Krasner MS, Quill TE, Suchman AL, et al. The impact of a program in mindful communication on primary care physicians. Acad Med. 2012;87(6):815–9. doi:10.1097/ACM.0b013e318253d3b2.
18. Hutchinson TA. Acknowledgements. In: Hutchinson TA, editor. Whole person care. A new paradigm for the 21st century. New York: Springer Science+Business Media, LLC; 2011.
19. Hutchinson TA, Mount BM, Kearney M. The healing journey. In: Hutchinson TA, editor. Whole person care. A new paradigm for the 21st century. New York: Springer Science+Business Media, LLC; 2011.
20. Cruess RL, Cruess SR. Whole person care, professionalism, and the medical mandate. In: Hutchinson TA, editor. Whole person care. A new paradigm for the 21st century. New York: Springer Science+Business Media, LLC; 2011.
21. Boudreau JD, Cassell EJ, Fuks A. A healing curriculum. Med Educ. 2007;41:1193–201.
22. Satir V, Banmen J, Gerber J, Gomori M. The satir model: family therapy and beyond. Palo Alto: Science and Behaviour Books; 1991.
23. Irving J, Park J, Fitzpatrick M, Dobkin PL, Chen A, Hutchinson T. Experiences of health care professionals enrolled in mindfulness-based medical practice: a grounded theory model. Springer Science+Business Media, LLC. Mindfulness. 2014;5(1):60–71.
24. Garneau K, Hutchinson T, Zhao Q, Dobkin P. Cultivating person-centered medicine in future physicians. Eur J Person Centered Healthc. 2013;1(2):468–77.
25. Hutchinson TA, Brawer JR. The challenge of medical dichotomies and the congruent physician-patient relationship in medicine. In: Hutchinson TA, editor. Whole person care. A new paradigm for the 21st century. New York: Springer Science+Business Media, LLC; 2011.
26. Satir V, Banmen J, Gerber J, Gomori M. The satir model: family therapy and beyond. Palo Alto: Science and Behaviour Books; 1991. p. 65–84. Chapter 4, Congruence.
27. Wald HS, Anthony D, Hutchinson TA, Liben S, et al. Professional identity formation for humanistic, resilient health care practitioners: pedagogic strategies for bridging theory to practice in medical education. Acad Med. 2015;90(6):753–60.

28. Satir V, Banmen J, Gerber J, Gomori M. The satir model: family therapy and beyond. Palo Alto: Science and Behaviour Books; 1991. p. 31–64. Chapter 3, The Survival Stances.
29. The Virginia Satir Global Network (producer). The Satir Family Series [10 DVDs].
30. Satir V, Banmen J, Gerber J, Gomori M. The satir model: family therapy and beyond. Palo Alto: Science and Behaviour Books; 1991. p. 19–30. Chapter 2, The Primary Triad.
31. Heath C, Heath D. Made to stick: why some ideas survive and others die. New York: Random House; 2007.
32. Watzlawick P, Bavelas JB, Jackson DD. Pragmatics of human communication: a study of inter-actional patterns, pathologies, and paradoxes. New York: W.W. Norton & Company; 1967. p. 48–71. Chapter 2, Some Tentative Axioms of Communication.
33. Whitney D, Trosten-Bloom A. The power of appreciative inquiry. A practical guide to positive change. 2nd ed. San Francisco: Berrett-Koehler Publishers; 2010.
34. McGill Programs in Whole Person Care. Mission Statement [Internet]. 2015 [cited 2015 July 14]. Available from: http://www.mcgill.ca/wholepersoncare/.

Chapter 5
Steps for Starting and Sustaining Programs

5.1 Introduction

Many people reading this book may have already begun to integrate mindfulness into the medical curriculum or are looking for ways to do that in the future. This process can be made easier or more difficult depending on how one goes about it. In this chapter, we will explore some key factors in how to do this successfully along with strategies on how to work with potential barriers.

5.2 Within a Medical School Curriculum

5.2.1 Aims and Objectives of Mindfulness-Based Programs

Whatever the level of integration, it is important to have reflected on what the program is aimed at doing and to make that explicit and clear to the students. Although the teaching of mindfulness can be seen as an open inquiry without defined aims, where each learner learns their own lessons in their own way and at their own pace, medical students and faculties are driven by definable, assessable, purposeful and achievable aims. Clear aims and objectives will avoid potential frustration and confusion and also shape the emphasis of the content and practices.

Although mindfulness is often spoken of as if it is one thing, it has many different aspects and applications. Programs can therefore vary enormously in their delivery, content and practical exercises depending on what applications are being emphasised. For example, a program with a major focus on self-care or stress management may utilise more contemplative exercises and the cognitive aspects of mindfulness. A program that has an emphasis on the role of mindfulness in enhancing communication may have more role-plays and clinical scenarios where the students experiment with being mindful while engaged in taking a history, or providing

© Springer International Publishing Switzerland 2016   65
P.L. Dobkin, C.S. Hassed, *Mindful Medical Practitioners*,
DOI 10.1007/978-3-319-31066-4_5

explanations or management for patients. There might be much more reflective conversation about empathy, picking up cues and body language.

Within one curriculum, the aims and objective may also be different at different stages of the medical course. For example, early in the course, the main aim may be fostering student self-care or understanding the basics of the mind-body interaction. Later in the curriculum, mindfulness teaching may move onto developing effective communication and motivational interviewing skills. Towards the end of the course, mindfulness teaching may move into developing high-level clinical reasoning skills, preventing clinical errors, managing the pressure of emergency situations or maintaining focus while engaged in complex medical procedures.

Aims and objectives can also be shaped by the amount of curriculum time available. If the time is limited, then the objectives may need to be more conservative. Better to do a few things well with some depth rather than trying to do too much and doing it poorly and superficially.

The particular aims and objectives for a mindfulness component of the course can also be shaped by what other elements of curriculum are being taught at the same time. If, for example, communication skills have not yet been introduced to the students, then exploring it at length in a mindfulness program may not make sense or be seen as relevant. If the students have not yet a sufficient depth of scientific understanding, then going into the mind-body relationship in too much depth may not be well understood. If students have not yet been exposed to clinical decision-making, then exploring cognitive bias may be seen as being of obscure importance.

Various applications of mindfulness programs have been explored in previous chapters, and the aims of some particular programs will be explored in more depth in Chap. 6.

5.2.2 Issues Related to Core Curriculum Versus Elective Programs

Running elective mindfulness programs is, relatively speaking, an easier prospect than programs embedded in core curriculum. In elective programs, students have self-selected to attend and are likely to be positively disposed to mindfulness before setting foot in the tutorial room. Perhaps they have recognised the need to manage their stress better, a desire to be more able to switch off from study concerns at night in order to sleep, or perhaps they have noticed how distractible they are when studying. They are more likely to have insight and motivation as to how mindfulness could help in such situations.

The main challenges with elective programs, however, are, first, adequately promoting the course to students. Second is finding funding sources and extracurricular time to run non-core course in already-packed curricula. Third is harnessing motivation for students to sacrifice time and engage with a subject for which they get no academic recognition. Out of hours, even motivated students are likely to battle with competing demands such as study, socialising and part-time employment. Initially, students may be motivated to come along, but when a mindfulness program competes with study demands for assessable components of the medical course, then they will often not attend, or at least not attend enough sessions to get significant benefit from it. The case needs to be clearly made to students that mindfulness may help with their more pressing priorities, for example, saving the students time by utilising study time in a more focused way or enhancing academic performance by reducing exam anxiety.

For mindfulness programs that are embedded as core curriculum, there are a different set of challenges. First, a case will have to have been made to the faculty in a much more rigorous way to make space for core mindfulness programs than for elective ones. Such a case needs to be based on a clearly argued, evidence-based rationale including student well-being, clinical needs and therapeutic potential. Second, half the students may step into the first mindfulness tutorial motivated and interested to varying extents, but the other half may be wondering why mindfulness is even in the curriculum perceiving it to be at the expense of topics more stereotypically associated with medical training like biomedical sciences. The case for mindfulness needs to be made to the students before getting to the experiential component. They need to have the rationale explained to them in language that is clinical, scientific and grounded and preferably by doctors or other respected health professionals. This is easy to do in large-group settings. Respected role models or patients describing their experience with mindfulness can also help in this regard. The students need to be made aware of the scientific basis of mindfulness and the accumulating evidence base underpinning it as well as the personal and professional cost to doctors of distraction and inattention.

All of this, to use a metaphor, is to get the horse to the water. The real learning about mindfulness obviously occurs when they drink, i.e. experience it. That the student must do for themselves. If the preparation and introduction to mindfulness is not done well, then students will not partake of the practice. To this end, the mindfulness tutor particularly needs skills in engaging motivation. This happens best by framing learning about mindfulness as an experiment to be tested and explored. Resistance and questions are welcomed when they arise, not opposed, all the while gently reframing healthy scepticism into further inquiry. The tutor needs to be able to elucidate the needs and interests of the various students in the room and to draw out why mindfulness might be relevant to them. As the weeks progress, it is what the students discover and share in the group that leads to the transformation. The tutor gently facilitates, helping the students to convince themselves through their own experiences and insights.

Especially in core-curricula programs, resistance needs to be handled carefully. Although mindfulness content may be assessable and therefore required learning, the students need to be clear that the personal practice of it is entirely their own choice. They may learn something by discussing their ambivalence to practising it or their oftentimes incorrect assumptions about it, but at the end of the day, the students are masters of their own ships. To impose it on students or become combative in the face of resistance is likely to entrench resistance, not reduce it. Furthermore, although mindfulness should be taught in a secular, practical and evidence-based way within a medical course, any reluctance to practicing it for religious reasons needs to be respected. Such resistance has been rare in the authors' experience, but such students can and should be directed to understand the clinical and scientific foundations of mindfulness and at least understand it in principle.

5.2.3 Contextualising It in the Curriculum

It is a great advantage to be able to plan the implementation of mindfulness-based teaching with a whole-of-curriculum view rather than taking an opportunistic or piecemeal approach where it is isolated to just one small part of the curriculum. A whole-of-curriculum view means being able to look at the curriculum overall and to see where mindfulness content would be most congruent with other course content and how to systematically and stepwise deepen students' understanding of mindfulness and how to apply it. An opportunistic or piecemeal approach to integrating mindfulness is better than not having it in the curriculum at all, but in this situation, a few hours of curriculum time here or there are given over to mindfulness teaching and then including whatever one can whether it is a good fit with other content or the students' level of development. This can make the teaching disjointed and hard to build up momentum and continuity.

Vertical and horizontal integration of mindfulness into the curriculum is important. As far as vertical integration is concerned, mindfulness teaching should be presented in such a way that students do not see it as repetition but rather as building upon and extending what has previously been learned. The intention is to take the students deeper and into applied mindfulness skills with an increasingly clinical focus. As far as horizontal integration is concerned, mindfulness teaching should never be seen as a separate subject disjointed from other core teaching especially the aspects of curriculum that medical students tend to take most seriously – the scientific, biomedical content and clinical skills.

If mindfulness programs are seen by students as peripheral to other elements of the curriculum, then its importance will be seen as marginal and as a 'soft' part of the course. For example, the Monash University curriculum is based on four themes: personal and professional development (e.g. self-care, ethics, law); health, knowledge and society (e.g. epidemiology, sociology, information management, evidence-based medicine); foundations of medicine (e.g. biomedical and psychological sciences); and clinical skills (e.g. communication, examination, procedural skills, motivational interviewing). Great care is taken to ensure that mindfulness content is made relevant to all themes. The introductory mindfulness lectures give a range of clinical scenarios, evidence and biomedical underpinnings of mindfulness and mind-body medicine. The mindfulness tutorials have role-plays of clinical scenarios where students are expected to respond to questions about mindfulness and recognise where it might be clinically relevant. It is integrated into communication skills tutorials and motivational interviewing, and students explore how mindfulness helps to foster empathy and compassion but reduce vicarious stress. Mindfulness is made relevant to self-care and stress management and how that impacts upon things like burnout and academic progress. It can be linked to ethics, compassion for others and acting with authenticity and self-awareness. In later years, it is linked to things such as clinical errors, decision-making and bias.

The broader integration of mindfulness is best done where it is mentioned, revisited and reinforced in other lectures or tutorials that are not labelled 'mindfulness teaching'. This requires that a wide number of faculty members understand and are sympathetic to mindfulness.

5.2.4 Presenting It to Faculty

Presenting mindfulness to the wider faculty can be done on a number of levels. To begin, it can be very helpful if as many faculty and clinical staff as possible have at least heard about mindfulness, perhaps being given an engaging and evidence-based presentation on it. At least as a result, they may understand and respect why it is or should be integrated into the curriculum. A number of faculty may want to go the next step of doing some basic mindfulness training to deepen their understanding and application of it. Some may want to go further and do training in order to teach mindfulness within the medical course. A skilful mindfulness teacher needs training in how to teach mindfulness as much as they need training in how to practice it. All of this plants the seed and helps to make the ground fertile for the growth of mindfulness.

If mindfulness is to be presented to the faculty as a new addition to the medical curriculum, or to expand it from a small existing base, then the case needs to be well made. If the ground has been previously prepared, then this job is a lot easier, but if very few have any knowledge about or experience of mindfulness, then resistance will potentially be more vocal. As was mentioned in relation to students, resistance can become more entrenched if it is opposed. It is best worked with in a gentle, non-confrontational manner where the arguments for it are simply and clearly put, supportive evidence provided and it is seen to complement and add value – not detract from and compete with – the other elements of curriculum.

Also important is the language that is used when speaking of mindfulness. If it is spoken of in terms that can be interpreted as mystical, spiritual or complex, or if Buddhist, Yoga or other philosophical language is used inappropriately, then it is likely to be seen as 'foreign' and rejected without due consideration. The rationale for mindfulness needs to be evidence based, secular and pragmatic as much as it needs to be faithful to the enduring philosophical principles underpinning it. The case needs to be made along similar lines to those which it was made relevant to students – self-care, effective communication, biomedical science, therapeutic benefits, enhanced decision-making, reduced errors, etc. If that is done well, then it is not so much a challenge to make a valid case for the inclusion of mindfulness, but rather the challenge is making a rational case that it shouldn't be included.

5.2.5   Faithful to the Philosophy but Flexible with the Form

Philosophical purists who learned mindfulness within spiritual contexts are likely to find it unsatisfactory if mindfulness is presented in pragmatic and scientific terms perhaps by faculty members who may not be deeply embedded within a spiritual path. It could reasonably be argued that this dilutes or debases mindfulness, but it could also be argued that to impose a philosophical agenda on it is inappropriate and potentially alienates many students who might otherwise have benefited from it. It needs to be remembered that a medical faculty is training doctors, not devotees. Students need to be met where they are. Their stated needs are practical and not spiritual, and the depth to which they are ready to explore and apply mindfulness is different to someone else who is looking for a deeper experience. Of course, if some wish to explore it more deeply, then they can do that in a way that is culturally, personally and spiritually congruent to them.

The philosophy underpinning its teaching needs to be faithful to its enduring principles. That doesn't mean that a mindfulness teacher must have extensive philosophical or spiritual insights into mindfulness – although it will undoubtedly help if they do. The proper training of faculty designing, delivering and overseeing mindfulness programs is vital lest what is being called mindfulness is something else entirely. Being flexible or lax with the philosophical underpinning of a mindfulness course can mean that it is misleading, loses its way and becomes ineffective.

Being faithful to the philosophy doesn't mean that one cannot be flexible with the form that the course takes. The form in which mindfulness is taught is infinitely variable, but it is easy to be rigid and inflexible regarding the form in which mindfulness is taught and therefore not be able to contextualise it effectively to the curriculum or adapt it to the amount of curriculum time available.

5.2.6   Making Mindfulness Examinable and How to Assess It

Assessment often drives learning. Such is the mentality of most medical students that the essential thing that drives what is or isn't worth learning is what is examinable. The depth that a medical student goes into a topic is likely to be strongly influenced by the number of marks allocated to that topic. Unfortunately, there are many things that are important but aren't assessed, or are very difficult to assess objectively, and are therefore seen as soft or peripheral to a medical students' interests. Many things are heavily assessed and are therefore seen as important by students, but years later, they will have long forgotten much of what they have learned as being irrelevant to the work of a doctor.

For mindfulness to be seen as a credible and an important part of the medical course, it needs to be assessable. This can be done in a number of ways. For example:

- Formative assessment:

  - For example, **reflective journals** outlining a student's personal experience as they progress through the mindfulness course. For such a journal to be authentic and useful as a reflective exercise, then it is preferable for it to be formatively (for learning) rather than summatively (for marks) assessed. If a reflective journal is summatively assessed, then students will generally write model rather than authentic reflections which are designed to impress the marker rather than be a credible account of the student's actual experiences. Even if a student doesn't engage with mindfulness meditation, there is still much they can reflect upon about the impact of inattention and distraction, the informal practice of being mindful, and the cognitive aspects of it.

- Summative assessment:

  - Written **essays** can be useful and deepen reflection significantly. The drawback is the potential burden on the students' time in writing them and faculty having to mark large numbers of them.
  - Questions on written **exams** such as multiple choice, extended match, short answer or short essay questions are important. They can test students' core knowledge of mindfulness and the mind-body relationship, the evidence and science supporting it, the clinical indications and contraindications for it or the principles of it. The presence of such questions on exams will significantly increase the students' engagement with the core content.
  - **OSCE stations**. Students might be required to communicate in a mindful or attentive way in general, but also to be able to communicate accurately about mindfulness itself, or to know when it would be appropriate to refer a patient for it in a clinical situation. For example, a standardised patient may be asking the student questions about it. Without more in-depth training, it would not be appropriate for a student to be expected to deliver a mindfulness-based intervention or lead a meditation practice.

There is a temptation not to make measurable the mindfulness content that appears in core curriculum, but we, the authors, believe that this is misguided. Yes, to some extent, it is counter to the philosophy of mindfulness to focus on an aim or outcome or to compel someone to learn about it. Assessment, therefore, should be focused on core knowledge and not on whether or not the student has personally practiced it, but if it is not assessable at all, then far fewer students will be motivated to practice, reflect and investigate it. Most will come away without even a theoretical understanding of it.

One other aspect of assessing mindfulness is to build in evaluation of the course and even link it to a research agenda. The prospect for randomised trials is not possible for programs integrated into core curriculum, but pre-/postcourse questionnaires can be provided as seen in Hassed et al. [1] and Garneau et al. [2]. These can also help students to monitoring their progress and potentially, if they wish, opt in to having their de-identified data included for educational research. It is important for faculties to measure if a program actually produces the benefits it professes to.

This can either confirm the case for mindfulness being included or, if a program is not meeting its stated aims, then raise questions as to why not.

5.3   Programs for Residents, Practicing Physicians and Allied Health Professionals

Many of the issues mentioned above for students are just as relevant for vocational programs for seasoned doctors and allied health professionals. It needs to have a context, a well-communicated rationale, be evidence based and assessable, be faithful to the philosophy of mindfulness and be in a form that is relevant and practical.

The maturity and clinical experience of postgraduates means that the depth of application is potentially greater, and clinical relevance is generally more obvious making it easier to engage them. On the other hand, the presence of already entrenched unmindful work habits can be a challenge.

Another challenge in vocational environments like hospitals is that although participants may want and need to attend a mindfulness course, they may find themselves unable to make time for it due to unceasing work demands, being on call and a work environment that values mindfulness training in principle but is less than accommodating in practice. To make it feasible to run a course within a hospital, there is a need to find cover for participants so that they can remove themselves from work commitments long enough to attend. This can be built into vocational training requirements through colleges. Attending weekend and evening courses may be an unattractive option for clinicians who already have very full rosters, but some may find it more workable than taking a course given over 2 months.

Although it is not uncommon that clinicians may think that a theoretical understanding of mindfulness is sufficient, it is vital to teach clinicians how to apply mindfulness with their patients by requiring them to first learn to apply it to themselves. In the process, they will gain personal benefit at the same time as they are developing a far deeper understanding of mindfulness.

5.3.1   CME Credits

To gain Continuing Medical Education credit, there is a need to apply to the relevant colleges and professional bodies. Just as the case needs to be made and contextualised for the presence of mindfulness within a medical curriculum, so too is there a need for the case to be made with clear and relevant learning objectives and appropriate assessment put in place.

It is also important to consider how mindfulness skills taught in a vocational course are going to translate to the work environment. For example, are medical insurers or government funders going to recognise the implementation of mindfulness in various clinical situations? Yes, particularly if there is good evidence for its use for that condition and that it is embedded as part of a total management approach. This is true, for example, in the United Kingdom where Mindfulness-Based Cognitive Therapy (MBCT) is covered under universal health care as first-line treatment for recurrent depression. If a briefer meditation practice is included in a consultation alongside counselling in an MBCT model or mindfulness is used as an adjunct for pain management, then it is not likely to be a problem. It may possibly be a problem when there is not enough evidence to support mindfulness' use for the condition under question or a one-on-one consultation is dominated by extended silent meditation practice in the absence of other medical or psychotherapies.

As more vocational medical education is being delivered in online formats, there is an understandable concern about whether it will be as effective as programs delivered face-to-face. The convenience of online delivery may come at a cost. There is not enough evidence to indicate how superior face-to-face-delivered programs are, but something significant is lost when there is no opportunity for reflection, dialogue and questions between an experienced mindfulness teacher and a practitioner receiving mindfulness training.

A clinician needs a far greater depth of understanding if they are applying mindfulness for significant mental and physical health problems than they might need if they are applying it for something less demanding. The clinician needs specific professional skills and experience in the chosen discipline along with in-depth mindfulness training.

5.3.2   Multidisciplinary Groups

The needs and applications for mindfulness training are similar for many allied health professionals as they are for doctors and doctors in training, although the emphasis may be different depending on the discipline. Students and practitioners from different disciplines learn from being trained together as their various perspectives enrich and inform a broader understanding of mindfulness.

A decade ago, McGill Programs in Whole Person Care launched a self-sustaining, self-funded, multidisciplinary program for doctors and allied health-care professionals. Physicians are offered 20 CME credits for full attendance (26 h). A description of a course in action on a week-by-week basis can be found in a book chapter entitled '*Mindfulness-Based Medical Practice: Eight Weeks* En Route *to Wellness*' [3]. For those that cannot attend an 8-week course, a weekend 14 h retreat is offered with ten CME credits. The groups are multidisciplinary.

For some clinicians, the end of the course marks the beginning of a lifelong practice for which they appreciate ongoing support. In 2011, a follow-up 'Living the Practice' course was launched by one of the authors (PLD). Participants are mostly physicians who wish to 'stay on track' and share experiences. They appreciate being part of a group of like-hearted clinicians. The materials covered and exercises originate from the teacher's ongoing continuing education.

References

1. Hassed C, de Lisle S, Sullivan G, Pier C. Enhancing the health of medical students: outcomes of an integrated mindfulness and lifestyle program. Adv Health Sci Educ Theory Pract. 2009;14:387–98. 2008 May 31. [Epub ahead of print] http://dx.doi.org/10.1007/s10459-008-9125-3.
2. Garneau K, Hutchinson T, Zhao Q, Dobkin PL. Cultivating person-centered medicine in future physicians. Eur J Pers Centred Healthc. 2013;1(2):468–77.
3. Dobkin PL. Mindfulness-based medical practice: eight weeks en route to wellness. In: Ivtzan I, Lomas T, editors. Mindfulness in positive psychology: the science of meditation and wellbeing. London: Taylor & Francis/Routledge; 2016. in press.

Chapter 6
Programme Delivery

Some of the principles and practicalities of introducing mindfulness programmes in medical education have been mentioned in previous chapters. This chapter will explore the principles of delivering such programmes and give examples of how some existing programmes in medical schools have gone about delivering their mindfulness content.

6.1 Part 1: Principles of Teaching Mindfulness to Medical Students and Doctors

6.1.1 Being Authentic and True to the Principles

In Chap. 5 with regard to starting mindfulness programmes, there was a discussion of the importance of staying faithful to the philosophy of teaching mindfulness but being flexible with the form in which it is taught. There are some further practical points to be made with regard to delivering those programmes. The key elements of learning and teaching mindfulness to remain faithful to are:

- Ensure that what is being called mindfulness is actually mindfulness.
- Mindfulness meditation, even if brief, is the cornerstone of learning to be mindful.
- The key cognitive aspects are mindful perception, non-attachment, acceptance, being non-judgmental, compassion to self and others and being in the present moment.
- Choose tutors carefully.
- Learning takes place through practice, experience, reflection and insight.
- There are no right or wrong experiences, only learning opportunities.
- Learning mindfulness is gradual and takes time.
- The first steps in applying mindfulness teach us how unmindful we tend to be.

© Springer International Publishing Switzerland 2016
P.L. Dobkin, C.S. Hassed, *Mindful Medical Practitioners*,
DOI 10.1007/978-3-319-31066-4_6

These key elements should be included in mindfulness programmes whether they be specific, overt learning objectives and teaching methodology or implicit principles underpinning what is taught and how it is taught.

Within a subject in a medical course, a variety of skills may be taught in conjunction with mindfulness, but if they are not consistent with mindfulness, then it is best to call it by another name. Sometimes the distinction needs to be nuanced. For example, forms of meditation that revolve around visualisation, affirmations or mantra meditation may not be considered mindfulness practices per se. Although they do involve the training of attention on an object (i.e. a thought or mantra), it would be better to label such practices as visualisation, affirmation or mantra-based practices. A further example might be that if students are being introduced to conventional Cognitive Behaviour Therapy, then there may be discussion about how mindfulness skills can complement and enhance it. If, on the other hand, the students are learning about hypnosis, then the distinction between mindfulness and this intervention needs to be clarified. Specifically, mindfulness is not a trance state, it does not involve the introduction of a particular thought or belief, and it does not aim to 'empty' the mind. Instead, it is non-elaborative and assists the person to impartially observe the thinking mind rather than elaborating on the thinking process.

Some well-known teachers of mindfulness, e.g. Ellen Langer from Harvard University, have long taught ways of being mindful that do not involve, or at least do not emphasise, the formal practice of meditation [1]. There are many ways of teaching mindfulness and many interpretations of what it means to be mindful. Some teachers who come to mindfulness from a deep commitment to extended formal meditation practice will stress that, but others will highlight that it can be cultivated equally well through informal practices. This balance needs to be struck correctly for the students' needs and level of commitment [2], but some contend that it is not really mindfulness if it does not include at least some practice of meditation.

Mindfulness is more than just meditation. It can be thought of as a way of being. The key cognitive aspects could be described and applied in a number of ways, but here are some suggestions: mindful perception, non-attachment, acceptance, being non-judgmental, compassion to self and others and being in the present moment. The main point to note here is that if what is being taught is not consistent with these – like being judgmental and reactive as a way of dealing with discomfort – then it should not be considered mindfulness.

Learning takes place not primarily through theory but through practice (apply meditation), experience (notice what takes place as it is applied), reflection (reflect on what arose from experience) and insight (learn the lesson underpinning that experience). Then, and only then, does the theory make sense. Every experience can teach us something, whether it is outwardly viewed as good or bad; this non-judgmental approach to learning is vital. It takes time for insight to arise; therefore developing patience is crucial. If, for example, a student in the first weeks of a programme comes to a realisation of how unmindful and distracted he or she is, then that is a sign of progress, not reason to be self-critical.

The final point about being authentic and true to the principles relates to teacher motivation, training and what they model for the students. This will be covered in Chap. 7.

6.1.2   Making It Practical and Relevant

Meet your students where they are. If you are not sure what is relevant to them, then you can ask or survey them – they will tell you. Their rationale for learning may be to study better, be less anxious, sleep better or transition more smoothly (e.g. from medical student to residency). Perhaps they are interested in learning strategies to help their patients with common problems. Do they wish to be more compassionate in how they respond to suffering, without getting overwhelmed by it? What is their agenda? An astute mindfulness teacher will be able to adapt the principles and practices of mindfulness for their needs.

One challenge can be to communicate to students why something like mindfulness is relevant when they have yet to encounter relevant situations. Perhaps they are not advanced enough in their courses or don't have enough clinical experience. In such situations it can help to have patients or respected clinicians explain why mindfulness matters to them. A patient may describe how fulfilling and reassuring it is to speak with a doctor who is communicating mindfully, or a neurosurgeon may relate how important it is to be vigilant and maintain focus during long and complex neurosurgical procedures. This can be done in a large-group format and is a valuable adjunct to preparing students for their small-group experiential learning.

6.1.3   Language

How something is said is often more important that what is said. If it is insensitively expressed, vague or in terms that are unfamiliar to the learner, then it will create resistance or may be seen as extraneous or foreign. A number of key aspects of language are briefly outlined herein.

First, keep it simple and linked to everyday experience students can readily relate to. Use common terms, or if using technical ones, translate them into simple and practical language. Demystify and avoid philosophical or spiritual ideology or terms.

Ensure that what is taught is inclusive and congruent to medical as well as ethnic cultures.

Metaphor, allegory, storytelling and sometimes poetry can be excellent ways of communicating concepts that are sometimes difficult to grasp or are paradoxical.

Mnemonics can be useful for remembering key points or steps involved in the practice of mindfulness.

Use inclusive language. For example, if a student is recounting a personal experience, respond in ways that invite everyone into the conversation and normalises experiences that could otherwise make a student feel isolated. For instance, 'So it seems that *we* have a mind that tends to wander off without us knowing' rather than 'So it seems that *you* have a mind that tends to wander off without you knowing'. This way of communicating reminds the teacher to be humble and actively engaged in the inquiry.

Speaking in the third person can help depersonalise otherwise personal experiences because it implicitly invites the person to take up the reference point of the impartial observer. For example, 'So what was observed taking place in *the* mind' is more likely to help the student look at mental activity in an impartial way than 'So what did you observe taking place in *your* mind'.

Also valuable is humour. A humorous aside, cartoon or anecdote can be instructive but also help to lower anxiety, maintain attention and foster openness. It is like the spoonful of sugar that helps the medicine to go down.

The tone of voice and response need to communicate mindful attitudes. If the teacher harbours a closed mind or a judgmental thought, then that will generally be communicated in the sound of the voice even though the teacher uses the 'right words'. This is one of the ways in which the teacher's mindfulness, or lack of, reveals itself.

6.1.4 Balance of Science, Theory, Philosophy and Practice

Medical or premed students are enrolled in a scientific discipline; thus, mindfulness needs to be taught as such, no less than any other part of the curriculum. If mindfulness is not presented as evidence based, it is easily dismissed or considered a 'soft' part of the curriculum.

The evidence and theory can engender interest and respect for mindfulness, but information *about* mindfulness is not the same as understanding it. Comprehension stems from experience and that is where the weight of curriculum time needs to be dedicated, following the theoretically and scientifically based introduction.

To ignore the philosophical basis of mindfulness could be a mistake. To fail to mention its roots could lead to a superficial or narrow understanding of it and runs the risk of disconnecting it from a deeper sense of what it means to be truly mindful. This issue will be covered in Chap. 8. On the other hand, if a passionate mindfulness enthusiast goes too far, or speaks too philosophically about it, this runs the risk of alienating a significant part of the student cohort. The majority may be interested in utilising mindfulness in pragmatic ways that are relevant for prospective doctors. They may be curious about a deeper backstory, as it were, but they can be quickly turned off if the exploration strays from what they consider safe and solid ground.

Receiving and taking note of student evaluations will assist in knowing whether that balance is being struck. If the significant number of students indicates that they are interested for more of a philosophical understanding, then offer more, but if there is pushback, then take note and determine where changes need to be made in content or how it is being taught.

6.1.5   Religious, Spiritual and Cultural Issues

As discussed in Chap. 5, it is important to emphasise that mindfulness be taught in a practical, grounded and secular way so it is seen as a universal practice and not belonging to any single group, religion or culture. Students who are non-religious tend to have their concerns or assumptions assuaged if it is presented in a secular manner. It is worth emphasising that although mindfulness has been well described and practised in Buddhist settings, so too have these attributes been well described in all wisdom traditions and cultures. There is nothing particularly eastern about it.

Religious or spiritual concerns about mindfulness are far less likely to be a problem if it is taught in such a way that it is personally and clinically focused and is supported by credible evidence. While mindfulness can be practised as a spiritual discipline, this is not why students are in medical school nor is it generally the reason that patients come to doctors seeking relief from their health-related problems.

In medical schools where introducing mindfulness has been done well, concerns are rare. Yet, if students are taught by someone who is evangelical or attempts to impose an ideology on them, then resistance is likely to arise.

For students who have a strong religious disposition, they may need to be reassured that they can practise of their own volition and in ways that are relevant to them. One student asked where mindfulness sat with his main spiritual discipline – prayer. He was questioned where his attention was when he was reciting his daily, well-rehearsed prayers. Was his attention fully with the prayer, or was he reciting the prayer on automatic pilot while his mind was thinking of other things? He reflected for a moment and recognised that he often prayed while on automatic pilot. The suggestion was then made that perhaps he might like to pray mindfully so that he could follow his much-valued spiritual practices but with greater devotion and attention. That suggestion made sense to him and he gained an insight that mindfulness is relevant to us whatever we are doing.

6.1.6   Working with Resistance

Working with resistance is not easy. In fact it can be one of the most challenging aspects for mindfulness teachers particularly in programmes embedded as core curriculum.

Opposing resistance can reinforce it and even entrench it. Arguing, explaining or justifying tends to be a less skilful means than gently welcoming resistance when it arises while directing the person towards a mindful inquiry. Doing this well starts with the teacher's attitude. If the teacher is attached to a particular 'positive' outcome, then resistance is potentially seen as threatening and will either be opposed or ignored. If the teacher is open and accepting, then he or she may find that resistance often has a question or assumption behind it that needs to be brought out into the open. That requires impartiality, interested inquiry and skills in dialectic exchanges.

Often such situations lead to the most illuminating insights or open up important questions that may lead to further inquiry not just for the individual who raised the issue but for the whole class.

If a student stubbornly refuses to engage with the mindfulness curriculum, perhaps because he or she has a closed mind or a significant misunderstanding about it, then that student still needs to have their point of view heard and respected. Nonetheless, he or she should not be allowed to dominate or negatively influence the class disrupting the learning process for the other students. This requires careful classroom management.

Resistance, especially if it is constant, very vocal or widespread, needs attention even though it might outwardly be dismissed as unreasonable. It will nearly always reveal something that the course designer or teacher needs to see and respond to. Perhaps the language is inappropriate, or the emphasis is wrong. Perhaps it does not have the right balance of science, clinical relevance and philosophy such that the students have not properly engaged with it. Whatever it may be, it needs attention, openness to feedback, necessary adjustments and reflecting on the outcomes of those changes. To conclude that the students just don't understand and remain stuck, doing the same thing, is likely to kindle more dissatisfaction.

6.2 Part 2: Variations for Programme Delivery

Research for this part of the chapter uncovered descriptions of programmes on websites or in manuals for the most part. We selected those with different formats rather than attempt to be exhaustive as our goal was to show how Mindful Medical Practice can be taught without being restricted to a particular framework (e.g. 8-week MBSR course). The programmes from Monash University, the University of Rochester and McGill University were described in Chap. 4 and are not repeated here. In the other universities we focus on here, some programmes are designed for residents, others for physicians and allied health-care professionals and one included educators and administrators as their target audience. Champions at the sites were interviewed to ensure accuracy and determine if changes have been made since the website went live.

6.2.1 Office of Resident Wellness, Faculty of Medicine, University of Toronto, Postgraduate Medical Education

Toronto is a major hub for mindfulness as Mindfulness-Based Cognitive Therapy was developed there along with researchers in the United Kingdom. Thus, it is not surprising that nine skill-based workshops from 1 to 2 h in length are offered to residents during academic half-days through the Office of Resident Wellness (ORW) at the University of Toronto. In addition, the ORW website offers links for guided meditation practices and videos relevant to Mindful Practice. They are taught by Mr. Hurst to groups of 10–25 participants. All are interactive, affording residents an opportunity to share experiences and interact with peers with the guidance of an experienced counsellor in the field of physician wellness. Importantly, programme directors endorse the activities and encourage their residents to attend. The learning objectives are:

1. To promote reflective group dialogue about common responses to the psychological, physical and emotional challenges faced by faculty and trainees
2. To broaden awareness of effective adaptive strategies and their link to quality of care
3. To provide training in self-regulatory practices that support faculty and trainees in enhancing well-being and performance

Ruetalo, Hurst and Edwards presented a poster based on 40 workshops presented to 16 postgraduate programmes with 272 participants (personal communication). Evaluations revealed that 88 % were satisfied or very satisfied with the workshops, and 92 % considered the content relevant to their work. The most valued aspects were the opportunity to reflect upon and discuss the topics, practical skills attained and knowledge gained. Barriers to uptake were named as well; these were insufficient time due to service demands to implement knowledge gained and personal limitations such as lack of motivation and fatigue. A few expressed discomfort sharing feelings in a group context.

The workshops are listed on the website and summaries are found below.[1]

- Enhancing Well-Being and Performance

  This skill-based workshop focuses on well-being and clinical performance strategies. The workshop draws from current research on self-regulation, expert behaviours and training for high stress environments. The format is interactive. Techniques taught include brief mindfulness techniques, solution-focused discussions and self-regulatory processes that enhance self-awareness, well-being and optimal performance during residency and beyond.
- Fatigue Management

  Drawing on a multidisciplinary approach to physical, cognitive, emotional and motivational fatigue, this introductory workshop outlines current knowledge and optimal strategies for managing the multiple factors that influence fatigue states. Countermeasures and strategies for improving sleep and alertness are covered. Experiential exercises for pre-sleep relaxation rituals and a repertoire of on-call tactics are offered to participants.

The four-part series covers the multifactorial aspects of fatigue in greater depth. Current knowledge about specific fatigue processes is presented, and participants

---

[1] http://www.pgme.utoronto.ca/content/wellness-workshop-series, accessed February 23, 2015; Interviewed Christopher Hurst, February 24, 2015.

are engaged in a discussion about key energy management strategies for each fatigue category:

Managing Sleep Deprivation and Physical Fatigue
   Managing Cognitive Fatigue
   Managing Emotional Exhaustion
   Managing Motivation

- Managing Transitions and Change throughout the Medical Career
  This interactive workshop uses a psychological model of transition to outline the inner challenges and adaptive changes that medical trainees frequently encounter during the training process. Through large and small group discussion, participants explore common challenges and coping strategies. A concrete plan for a sustainable approach to self-care necessities and successful anticipation of transition phases is then developed.
- Mindful Career Planning
  Through reflection, discussion and self-assessment, residents are led through an interactive enquiry examining their projected career paths and the many influences that may impact career planning. The goal is to develop a framework for understanding how to make meaningful career decisions at pivotal points throughout their professional lives. This workshop draws heavily on the module developed by Dr. Susan Lieff for the RCPSC CanMEDS Manager Train-the-Trainer curriculum.
- Enhancing Exam Preparation and Performance
  Preparing well for OSCEs and written exams requires a multilevel approach that includes awareness of pacing, peak attentional periods, optimal studying practices and priorities and clear strategies for enhanced performance before and during exams.
- Time Management
  This interactive workshop provides a framework for effective time management, encourages residents to reflect on fundamental priorities in order to make mindful decisions about how they choose to use the limited time they have and provides opportunities to discuss and apply specific time management strategies.
- Resident Resilience in the Context of Adverse Events: A Mindful Approach
  Resident resilience is discussed in the context of adverse events, professional roles and personal reactions. Videos, group discussion and storytelling exercises are employed to open up the subject of adverse events for discussion, reflection, self-care planning and professional responsibility.
- Mindfulness in Medical Life: Focusing on Attentional Skills Development for Well-Being and Performance
  This workshop is primarily a skill-based and experiential approach to learning and integrating mindfulness skills into both personal and professional aspects of a medical life. The workshop offers a brief overview of contemporary research into mindfulness skills and their documented effects on well-being and cognitive and perceptual performance. A conceptual framework for developing mindfulness in medical practice to improve decision-making and patient care is outlined.

- Downward Docs: Mindful Yoga and Medicine
  This interactive and highly experiential workshop focuses on mindfulness, mindful movement, physical awareness and group reflection and discussion. The workshop offers an introduction to mindfulness concepts, basic yoga sequences and attentional skills related to movement and breath. Research evidence supporting the application of mindfulness and yoga in medical training is presented. The workshop concludes with a discussion on integrating mindfulness and breath work into residents' personal and professional lives. The instructors for the workshop are both certified yoga teachers and physicians.

6.2.2   University of Wisconsin Family Medicine Residency

The University of Wisconsin is recognised internationally for its research on mindfulness; thus, it is a natural extension to find clinical applications there. According to the website,[2] family medicine residents partake in a series of integrative medicine and self-care-related lectures entitled, 'Aware Medicine' over the course of the 3 years of family medicine residency training. In the context of integrative medicine, mindfulness is embedded along with other topics covered in whole person care such as the role spirituality plays in health, healing and cultural sensitivity. The website offers self-awareness exercises (e.g. a survey 'How Healthy Are You?' completed online) and self-care resources. Residents are directed to the website and encouraged to learn on their own. Monthly 'check-in' groups led by faculty and teachers from the University of Wisconsin Mindfulness Center are offered during resident seminar times. These are optional. The 'check-ins' begin with a brief meditation and then cover various topics related to resident well-being. Sessions may involve body scans, yoga and group discussions on mindful awareness with the intention of teaching the residents self-care and giving them tools to use with their patients as well. Trainees are guided in making the transition into being an attending physician and adjusting to their roles and responsibilities. Mentors are available for further one-on-one guidance in self-care, spirituality and mindfulness training. Retreats are available in the community. Some are silent retreats, while others promote Mindful Medical Practice. A description of one resident's experience is found in Minichiello [3].

Fortney et al. [4], a group from the University of Wisconsin, Department of Family Medicine, published a paper describing an abbreviated MBSR programme for 30 primary care clinicians (87 % were physicians). What is of interest here is how they modified the programme to suit the schedules of the participants. It was 18 h (rather than 29–33 h), run for 3 h on Friday evening, 7 h on Saturday and 4 h on Sunday with two follow-up sessions in 2 h evening time slots. The content was

---

[2] www.fammed.wisc.edu, accessed January 13, 2015; Dr. Vincent Minichiello, PGY2 was interviewed on February 17, 2015.

similar to standard MBSR programmes but less home practice was assigned (10–20 min of meditation, rather than 45 min/day). A website was designed specifically to help clinicians bring their Mindful Practice into the examination room. During class time, the clinicians were encouraged to share examples of applying mindfulness to their practice, i.e. working with patients using attitudes such as patience, non-judgment and empathy. Pre- to post-programme data showed improvements on burnout, stress, depression and anxiety scores with no significant changes on resilience or compassion scores, which were high to start. These benefits were maintained for 9 months.

6.2.3   Online Courses and Support Materials

The digital age has led many who wish to learn about mindfulness and integrate it into their work and personal lives to turn to the Internet. This enables those who cannot attend workshops or courses for various reasons (lack of funds, time, mobility or proximity to teaching centres) an opportunity to begin or continue learning. In fact, many sites provide links to genuine teachers, lectures and handouts. Yet, there is a risk that the person may be deterred by the sheer number of sites and lack of knowledge regarding how to select one. Moreover, the social fabric woven into classes where participants, led by a facilitator, often work in dyads and small groups is hard, if not impossible, to reconstruct in such a forum. While audiotapes of guided meditation practices can be downloaded for free and videos can be viewed at any time, the person is left to his or her own devices. Without a teacher or group with whom to exchange, if motivation wanes or the learner experiences confusion, she/he may simply be discouraged and give up. Many who take an MBSR course indicate that they tried to learn on their own but found that they needed a teacher the structure of a class and the support inherent when with others. Turning to the Internet, rather than other people in real time, underscores aspects of modern Western culture that may perpetuate feelings of alienation and isolation. If by doing so the person is seeking a quicker, easier path that can be taken 24/7, then this may reflect part of the problem that is leading the person to the Internet to begin with. That being said, for a person who is firmly grounded in mindfulness practice, certain sites may be beneficial for ongoing study and personal development. Or, when materials are posted as part of a class, then this can be expedient.

For example, the University of Ottawa Medical School launched a course for second year medical students. Their website[3] is used in conjunction with this course; it offers an e-book, *Mindfulness for Medical School, Residency, and Beyond*, written by Dr. MacLean a neurologist and content director of the mindfulness curriculum. Students are asked to read the book and view posted videos as part of their homework (e.g. 'Mindfulness reduces physician burnout', by Dr. Krasner). These materials are

---

[3] http://www.uofomindfulness.com, accessed February 13, 2015; Dr. MacLean was interviewed on January 29th, 2015.

used in class led by clinician-teachers who have sought their own mindfulness train-ing personally; they are not, however, trained at the University of Ottawa Medical School to do so.[4] The first class is mandatory for the medical students and seven other non-mandatory classes are offered; each is 1 h long. A half-day workshop on mind-fulness is integrated into the family medicine rotation when they are in the third year clerkship. Electives on mindfulness are available to all first and second year medical students.

Other attempts at a 'hybrid training model' have been made. For example, Kemper and Yun [5] combined an online course available for free with a small group ($n = 7$) of medical students led by a resident who 'has some prior meditation experience but was not formally trained as a MBSR facilitator'. They met for 1 h for 8 weeks to discuss the material; a Facebook page was available for 'group discus-sion' as well. Given that attendance was not good (one dropped out, most attended half of the classes) and only half completed the pre- post-course online question-naires, it seems that this model was not supported even though the authors suggested otherwise.

6.2.4   McMaster Programme for Faculty Development: Faculty of Health Sciences

While this work is highlighted in Chap. 8, we briefly describe courses designed for administrators, managers and a broad range of clinical faculty including doctors (about 25 % who take the courses), nurses and social workers. These descriptions below were written by Dr. Frolic and her colleagues and are reprinted with permis-sion.[5] The format differences are shown with italics:

- MBSR Adapted for Health-Care Professionals (based on the University of Massachusetts Center for mindfulness programme)
  This *standard 8-week course* for 20–25 participants (with 28 h of contact, 2 h classes over 10 weeks and a full day silent retreat) focuses on self-discovery and personal resilience through experiential learning, including a variety of mindfulness meditation practices and reflective exercises. Most class time is devoted to meditation, as well as small and large group discussion of the appli-cation of mindfulness to daily life and at work. Themes relevant to health care such as, mindful communication, mindful leadership are added to make it useful for participants who work in various health care settings. Home assignments (15–30 min each) are integrated into the course and a 'buddy system' is added to encourage practice.
- Mindful Communication (based on the University of Rochester School of Medicine and Dentistry model)

---

[4] The issue concerning teacher training will be covered in Chap. 7.

[5] Dr. Frolic was interviewed on February 18, 2015.

This course focuses on enhancing communication and integrating mindfulness in the workplace through deeper engagement with stories. This is facilitated through experiential learning, including a variety of mindfulness meditation practices, as well as reflective exercises using Appreciative Inquiry, Narrative Practice and Insight Dialogue. The goal, in addition to individual well-being, is to develop the facility to apply these skills spontaneously in a variety of contexts. This *year-long course* for 20–25 participants (53 h of contact *over 19 meetings*) is useful to those seeking a community to support their efforts at integrating mindfulness into clinical practice, teaching and leadership.

- Discovering Resilience Through Applied Mindfulness (based on the Factor-Inwentash Faculty of Social Work at the University of Toronto, Canada)
  This course focuses on increasing participants' understanding of the *neuroscience of mindfulness* and enabling *personal and organisational transformation* through mindful and compassionate action (*secular ethics*). Due to the large-group format (60–80 participants), lecture-style teaching is interspersed with experiential meditations, reflective exercises and group discussions. Two or three teachers co-lead the course. The intensive, immersion-style format [64 contact hours offered over *8 full days, one weekend (Friday and Saturday) each month for 4 months*], lends itself to community-building by including catered lunches. Participants develop working knowledge of the neuroscience of attention, cognition, self-regulation, relationship and research on interdisciplinary mindfulness.
- Transforming Compassion Fatigue (based on the work of Françoise Mathieu M.Ed., CCC. Director of Compassion Fatigue Solutions Inc.)
  This experiential 3 h workshop for 15–20 participants provides a brief introduction to a range of strategies for enhancing resilience. Participants learn about the impact of working in health care, learn to identify signs and symptoms associated with compassion fatigue and explore self-care strategies including mindfulness to help mitigate the impact of the work. Participants engage in reflective exercises to begin to identify a plan to stay healthy while working in health care.
- Narrative Health Care (based on the literature on narrative medicine)
  This 3 h workshop focuses on the skills required to enhance the development narrative competence – the ability to better communicate and work empathically with the stories patients bring. Using the skills of reflective writing and close reading, the workshop demonstrates the importance of not forcing the patient's illness narrative into the biomedical model but rather allow for the telling of the story from the patient's perspective.

What is most interesting at McMaster is that gradually the culture of care is being transformed by including hundreds of health-care personnel in one of these programmes or workshops. The story behind this successful endeavour will be summarised in Chap. 8. It is included in this book because we recognise that until the decision makers for education and clinical work understand the relevance of Mindful Medical Practice, it is unlikely that it will be integrated into the daily work lives of physicians, residents, medical students and allied health-care professionals. In other words, if the new behaviours consistent with mindfulness are not reinforced, or worse – are extinguished, then individuals taking these courses will default to what they are rewarded for even if it costs them their health and the opportunity to foster healing in their patients.

For example, an invitation to teach an 8-week Mindful Medical Practice to family medicine residents working in an economically depressed part of Montreal, Canada, where their patients typically presented with as many social problems as health issues arose because the director of their residency programme had taken the 8-week programme himself. He thought it would be helpful for his residents, especially since many were on disability/burnout leave. The residents were allowed 'protected time' to take the course and were provided with a catered meal before each evening class. What was not expected was that eight supervisors requested to join the group. While this could have been a problem, in that those higher up in the hierarchy would be privy to what was shared during the classes, it turned out that their participation enabled them to be supportive of the 12 residents who took the course when they adapted how they treated patients and took better care of themselves.

This thorny issue of hierarchy in medicine and mindfulness is the subject of a paper describing MBSR taught to a mixed group of doctors and patients in Paris, France – a society known for its entrenched social structure [6]. What occurred as the doctors became more self-aware and opened to the personhood of the patients in the group was that they were able to listen more deeply to others and became more compassionate towards themselves and others.

References

1. Langer E. Mindfulness. 25th anniversary edition. Boston: De Capo Press; 2014.
2. Hassed C. Training the mindful health practitioner: why attention matters. In: Le A, Ngnoumen CT, Langer EJ, editors. The Wiley Blackwell handbook of mindfulness. Chichester: Wiley; 2014. doi:10.1002/9781118294895.ch32.
3. Minichiello V. Finding my voice in residency. Reflections on integrative family medicine. Int J Whole Person Care. 2015;2(2):37–40.
4. Fortney L, Luchterhand C, Zakletskaia L, Zgierska A, Rakel D. Abbreviated mindfulness intervention for job satisfaction, quality of life, and compassion in primary care clinicians: a pilot study. Ann Fam Med. 2013;11(5):412–20. doi:10.1370/afm.1511.
5. Kemper KJ, Yun J. Group online mindfulness training: proof of a concept. J Evid Based Complement Altern Med. 2015;20(1):73–5. doi:10.1177/2156587214553306.
6. Dobkin PL, Bagnis CI, Spondenkiewicz M. Being human in medicine: beyond hierarchy. Int J Wholes Person Care. 2015;2(1):38–49.

Chapter 7
Educating Teachers

Do not try to satisfy your vanity by teaching a great many things. Awaken people's curiosity. It is enough to open minds, do not overload them. Put there just a spark. If there is some good inflammable stuff, it will catch fire [1].

7.1 Important Considerations

What is education? It seems like a simple question but considering the etymology of the word 'education', a less obvious but more interesting answer emerges. Education originates from the Latin word, *educare*, which means *to draw out*. It is not a matter of filling the students' minds with facts, although for certain purposes this is necessary. Education as a 'drawing out' implies there is wisdom and insight within the student that can be uncovered. The curiosity associated with an open and inquiring mind is the instrument essential for that search. Unfortunately, all too often, the emphasis on memorising information stifles interest.

Who then is the teacher? In light of the real meaning of education it must have something to do with the teacher being able to foster wonder, curiosity and an inquiring mind. This is consistent with cultivating a mindful attitude. Teaching mindfully aims to do just that. McCowen et al. [2] stress the importance of the 'who' in this basic question. They contend that the person teaching can inspire others to live fully in the moment, accept life as it presents itself and thrive as a consequence if the instructor practises what she/he teaches (not preaches). The three key characteristics of this person are (a) being authentic, (b) having authority and (c) offering friendship. Together these characteristics reflect integrity and care. The first entails being the person who has lived, loved and lost such that when interacting with others, there is a sense that the instructor is reality based or 'grounded'. Even such an authentic teacher's mistakes are an opportunity to serve as a fallibility model for the student by drawing out the learning from such experiences. It takes humility to teach in such a way but those who do accelerate learning [3] by

© Springer International Publishing Switzerland 2016   89
P.L. Dobkin, C.S. Hassed, *Mindful Medical Practitioners*,
DOI 10.1007/978-3-319-31066-4_7

making it easier for the student to acknowledge and learn from their own mistakes rather than conceal them. The second implies that the instructor knows what she/he knows because she/he has lived, examined, integrated and internalised it. Authority encompasses professional identity, training and skills – to be elaborated upon later in this chapter. As for friendship, relationships are founded on mutual respect, trust and recognition that each individual is capable of uncovering what they need to discover. It acknowledges that the teacher and student are there for the same reason or on the same team in contributing to the well-being of others. Such a teacher embodies compassion which is central to medicine's *raison d'être*. They create an atmosphere of psychological safety in which the learner is free to pose questions without the threat of being made to feel inadequate or foolish. Mindfulness-based teachers are guides on a path towards healing and wholeness, not fixers of broken people.

Not knowing what is 'best' for others, the teacher invites them to explore and find their own answers. Thus, the teacher puts his/her professional role, such as physician who prescribes medications, in the background and places his/her facilitator/teacher role in the foreground. This does not mean that the former role should be discarded as it may be needed should a situation arise that requires more direct action. For example, if working with a participant who was traumatised in the past and suddenly begins to cry uncontrollably in the group setting, the teacher-therapist would know how to help the person explore the emotions (as a therapist would) while inviting the group to witness and bear the person's suffering with compassion.

In order to be a teacher who can encourage others to find their way, the same attitudes that are fostered in mindfulness practice apply to the instructor. She/he needs to be curious and open-minded, flexible, non-judgmental, patient, kind, able to regulate his/her own emotions and switch between *doing* to *being* modes. A mindful teacher takes a different stance than that of the expert or problem solver. She/he 'leads from behind' in the sense of being a facilitator, a co-explorer and a questioner rather than being merely an instructor. A qualitative study conducted in the Netherlands in which participants and teachers in a Mindfulness-Based Cognitive Therapy course were interviewed and participated in focus groups confirmed the value of these qualities [4]. Specifically, four overarching themes were uncovered: the importance of embodiment, empowerment, non-reactivity and peer support. Mindful teachers were compassionate and used language that encouraged participants to adopt a non-patient role. Thus, there was less emphasis on hierarchy. These findings were reflected in a study conducted in France where MBSR was taught to three groups: one for patients, one for clinicians and one for a mix of doctors and patients [5]. While each has their own identity, hierarchy was dismantled in the third group explicitly and implicitly in the other two groups. Clinicians and patients interacted as equals. Participants with chronic illness were aided in discarding the heavy cloak of a diagnosis – one that contributed to their being overidentified with their illness (e.g. 'I am a diabetic'). Instead, they were seen as individuals who happened to be living with a medical condition and needed help from another person who could guide him or her accordingly.

7.2 Teachers' Skills

McCowen [6] describes four essential skills vital to teaching mindfulness-based programmes:

1. Stewardship – the teacher creates a unique learning environment.
   While the group is not seen as a type of psychotherapy or peer support group, group processes unfold and an effective teacher understands these dynamics. The teacher is explicit from the first class on that there is freedom of expression and all are invited to speak their truth. Everyone (including the teacher) is discouraged from giving advice or trying to solve anyone else's problems. The teacher summons all to participate without pressuring those who learn vicariously, say little or nothing at all. Over time the participants begin to feel that they belong to the group.

   When the group is run well, there is a sense of resonance. Most importantly, groups are led in a manner that is non-hierarchical, non-pathologising and non-instrumental. The message is since there is more right than wrong with you, there is no need to strive to change although as awareness grows, insight grows, and as a result change happens of itself. The teacher accepts that his or her role will seem to diminish over time because the participants become more active and gain confidence as their practices deepen.

2. Homiletics – the teacher engages with and responds to the group.
   Simplicity is the hallmark of expertise. Thus the teacher needs to be so familiar with the material being conveyed that it is expressed simply, practically and in a way that can be related directly to personal experience. As an example, when examining how stressful events impact the mind, body and emotions, this is explained with the aid of diagrams provided in the home practice workbook that are easy to follow. Participants are asked to provide examples of how this is true for them. One may note that work deadlines trigger a migraine headache; then the teacher would help the person examine if thoughts and emotions are linked to this physiological reactivity.

3. Guidance – the teacher helps others learn.
   The use of language is precise and purposeful. To guide a meditation practice, the instructor needs to use clear language that reflects mindfulness – staying in the present moment, accepting what emerges and working with it skilfully. The instructor invites, allows and guides while keeping the themes to be conveyed in mind. She/he listens for participants' words that reflect striving, doing, fixing and dualism and is careful not to project the idea, 'I am experienced so I will show you'. The mindful instructor acknowledges that we all, student and teacher alike, are a 'work in progress'. She/he guides by being connected to his/her own experience, such as awareness of breath, while teaching.

4. Inquiry – an open-ended look into direct experience.
   Crane et al. [7] refer to inquiry skills as 'disciplined improvisation'. This echoes Epstein's [8] description of engaging in Mindful Practice as if you were playing a musical instrument – you listen, feel and respond concomitantly. Much like a

musician, the teacher needs to practise (scales/meditation) diligently, observe and receive feedback from an 'accomplished' teacher in order to conduct inquiry adroitly. Inquiry involves the teacher leading the person through an exploration of his or her experiences of formal and informal mindfulness practices as well as weekly home assignments. When done well through modelling mindful inquiry, the student becomes an astute but impartial observer of their own experience and gains an accepting but interested attitude towards events as they unfold. Since this exchange takes place in a group setting, others in the room learn in various ways such as exploring similarities or differences from the person speaking. How the dialogue evolves is crucial and complex. The student is supported by the teacher's mindful attitudes (e.g. non-judgmental, curious) and led to the real-isation that what one notices in practice applies to the themes of the course, work and life in general. Conditioned habits (e.g. eating compulsively) and unhealthy mind states (e.g. self-critical thoughts) may be brought into awareness. Inquiry requires cultural sensitivity and emotional intelligence such that the student feels safe and free to explore. Importantly, the teacher is just as interested in and wel-coming of what a student could view as 'negative' experiences as they are of the 'positive' ones. A student might think, for example, that she/he is getting it wrong if she/he can't clear his/her mind or stop thoughts from coming in, but if such an experience is explored mindfully, then there is much to learn from it. The main aim is learning through insight not 'getting it right', and if this is done mindfully, then there are no positive or negative experiences; there are simply learning experiences and each is as valuable as the next. Students who are preoc-cupied about getting things right may not share what is going on for them or might try to change their experience in such a way to make it look right in the eyes of the teacher or other classmates. What the teacher and the group need is to hear things described as they are – authenticity is paramount to learning.

An example from a workshop offered by Hickman, Ucok and Krasner 'Rhetoric, Rhythm and the Rest Between Two Beats: Conversation Analysis as a Profound Teaching in Mindfulness' [9] characterises this process (what is written in CAPS represents comments on the exchange):

P: Participant
S: Sam (teacher)

P: Uhm, I am having a terrible time. I um I had a practice in the past and that's kind of falling apart. And I came to this hoping that I would kind of reconnect with my practice myself, and I'm just having a terrible time it's just not coming (NEGATIVE ASSESSMENT)
S: What's your name?
P: Sandra
S: Sandra
P: Yes
S: Well thank you
S: Sandra, could you say a little bit more descriptively what terrible means? (START OF THE INQUIRY; PROBE FOR MEANING)

P: Uhm

S: What do you notice? (ASKS ABOUT THE EXPERIENCE)

P: (outbreath with sound)

S: What is your experience? (MORE SPECIFIC; STAYS IN THE PRESENT MOMENT)

P: I notice I'm bored; I notice I'm impatient; I notice I'm distracted; I notice I feel like a failure [up to this point, her voice is slightly shaky and sad]

P: That sounds pretty awful [smiling tone]

S: That's up to you (DOES NOT CONFIRM OR REJECT)

S: So, so far we know that you: notice boredom impatience, distractibility, the feeling of failure (FORMULATION; GETS THE GIST OF IT)

P: Hm-hu and also I can't decide anything; I can't decide if I wanna be with people; I don't wanna be with people; I wanna walk in the sun if I wanna walk in the shade

S: Hm

S: And is that driving you crazy?

P: Uhm mm-uh huh huh I think it is crazy

S: So, have you heard in the meditation instructions suggestions that you shouldn't be bored or impatient or distracted or any of that? Or have you heard any instructions about how we suggest you work with the judgments around for instance being a failure? (GUIDES HOW TO EXPLORE THE EXPERIENCE)

P: Yes

S: And what have you noticed? What do you know about what we said about boredom and impatience and distractibility?

P: Just to notice it to stay with it to be with it

S: Right, so if that's the case, I mean that doesn't necessarily mean it's so

S: That it actually has perturbed you to the point of saying, I'm failing at this

P: Hh well part of it I think is being bored and impatient and distracted (JUDGMENT). And not in that place that I want to be. I feel like um it's a waste of time. Why am I doing this?

S: Yes, exactly so you have a memory of how it - how it ought to be or this place where you could be (AFFIRMATION AND SECOND FORMULATION)

P: U-hu

S: But it's not here. Right?

S: Is what you're saying? (SEEKS TO VERIFY)

S: Not the way you imagined. It's not-

P: Its not now: A-ha (INSIGHT)

S: And the instructions have a lot to do with now

S: True?

P: Right

S: So what's the problem?

P: I hate it (smiling tone). I wanna go home [smiling tone further emphasised]

S: Thank you

S: So if we could resume; can we go on? (SEEKS PERMISSION)

P: Sure

S: So you just really described that it doesn't feel good; so you'd rather not be in that place is that correct?

P: That's correct

S: Yea so that's part of what I was speaking about doing the practice. Since you have reported that you had practice in the past and you know

S: Something about the mind's tendency to not be where it actually is. So boredom and restlessness are flipsides of the same experience which is, I don't wanna be where I am (PERSONAL CONTEXT OF UNDERSTANDING EXAMINED)

P: Hhhum (slight sound with outbreath)

S: Like two sides of the same coin and so it may be an interesting exploration to: notice just how much that impulse comes up to – to hate it as in, I don't wanna be where I am, and to see if you can begin slowly with a lot of patience or at least kindness…

P: Hmm

S: To open to what is here now over and over and over again and it won't necessarily be a smooth incline but it will have its own kind of rises and falls and ebbs and flows and peaks and valleys simply make that your practice and that's what I meant about honouring whoever arrives so what's arrived lately is boredom and impatience and distractibility and I don't like it and all of that is okay except it doesn't feel okay but that's ultimately part of the practice; it is other than the practice you might consider doing yourself an interesting favour which is not spending too much time wishing you were back in that quiet state that you used to be because you might never return there and be better off for it 'cause that's just what was – rather than what is unfurling now we have an interesting way of creating cages and prisons that keep us where we're most comfortable; what we are most familiar with rather than a sort of larger familiarisation with a much bigger world, bigger sense of who it is that I am, who I may be (SUMS UP AND POINTS TO A UNIVERSAL CONCEPT THAT THE GROUP MAY RELATE TO)

The reader may notice that in general, there are layers in inquiry.[1] Layer 1: the teacher asks about sensations, thoughts and feelings. Layer 2: the teacher helps the person explore via direct noticing within a personal context of understanding. Layer 3: the teacher encourages exploration of what was learned via the first two layers for the person and the group. The teacher may wish to ask permission before delving into the depths with participants, sensing when it is appropriate and asking open-ended questions (e.g. how did bringing awareness to this experience affect it?). Implicit in the whole process is that the teacher asks the questions and the student gives the answers. This is *educare*.

In Crane et al.'s [10] study, the first to observe and analyse themes revealed in inquiry, they described:

- Turn-taking talk involving questions and reformulations
- Development of patients' skills in describing direct experiences
- Talk that fostered connection and affiliation within the group

---

[1] The author (PLD) acknowledges Dr. Patricia Luck's handout provided at the University of Rochester Advanced workshop given in 2015.

The student's language is shaped by the teacher towards the norms of mindfulness (e.g. to reinforce the perspective of the impartial observer, one speaks of 'the' mind, rather than 'my' mind). The teacher purposely turns to the others in the room to investigate whether the student's experience is similar such that they are included in the exchange. McCowen [6] emphasises a process called 'co-creation'. Inquiry is like a carol being sung in a choir – it is derived from both the sheet music (class plan) and the voices of the group from moment to moment.

Other important aspects of mindful inquiry include 'panning back', 'validation' and 'keeping a question open'. Panning back is like a camera zooming out from the detail of a scene to the larger view or perspective. It refers to group participants being invited to share personal experiences. On one level these experiences are particular to that individual but the teacher is interested in what lesson or principle can be learned from it. If the inquiry heads in this direction, then something of universal importance is discovered. The singular is an opportunity to illustrate the universal. This contrasts with what happens when students merely share personal experiences without inquiry. Self-disclosures may become occasions to vent negative emotions, but rarely is this useful. Validation is important and typically takes place at the end of the inquiry; the teacher may underline or sum up the lesson that has been distilled from the exchange. If, however, a question is not resolved in one inquiry, it is prudent for the teacher to keep it open for further exploration during the week. Often members of the group return in the following weeks with novel insights and experiences that shed light on the question. This fosters the spirit of inquiry and circumvents the temptation for the teacher to 'give the answer' or come to a quick and hasty resolution of an issue.

A consensus is developing with regard to requisite skills. These are:

- Confidence leading meditation practices and inquiry in a group setting
- Capacity to create an environment that supports reflection and dialogue
- Experience working within a health-care setting such that first-hand knowledge of the challenges and hardships inherent in them
- Familiarity with informal practice of mindfulness
- First-hand experience of applying mindfulness in the work setting

Crane et al. [10] describe the aptitude to toggle between being and doing modes. A teacher in the being mode is described as:

- Recognising and describing direct experience
- Being in touch with direct sensory perception moment by moment
- Approaching internal and external experience non-judgmentally
- Letting go of agendas and ambitions

Whereas a teacher in the doing mode is described as:

- Understanding and articulating rationales for processes
- Connecting direct experience with conceptual understandings
- Having a clear curriculum as a foundation for the programme
- Basing clinical programmes and curriculum choices on a clear rationale and evidence-based underpinnings
- Measuring outcomes routinely to check efficacy

The reader is encouraged to examine McCowen's [6] multidimensional model for an informative perspective on the dimensions of doing and non-doing. He proposes the three 'Cs' of doing: corporeality, knowing through the body; contingency, which recognises the impermanence of everything; and cosmopolitanism, the quality to allow meaning to emerge from the group exchanges. Within the non-doing dimension, he stresses the importance of non-pathologising, non-hierarchical and non-instrumental, i.e. 'non-actions'. These are all taking place within the dimension of friendship – a 'we-centric' space that is relational by nature.

7.3   Training Programmes

Many training programmes exist; herein we highlight a few select examples.

7.3.1   University of Massachusetts Medical School Center for Mindfulness

Oasis, housed at the University of Massachusetts Medical School Center for Mindfulness (CFM) in Medicine, Health Care, and Society has been a pioneer in training MBSR teachers. They maintain that to become a teacher, you need to devote time and energy to your psychological development and maintain a regular meditation and body-based practice such as yoga and attend silent retreats. Teachers need to have a professional training and a graduate degree in a related field (psychology, education, medicine). To become an MBSR teacher involves steps that are sequenced.

First, one participates in a 7-day MBSR residential retreat as a learner. The theoretical, philosophical and pedagogical underpinnings of MBSR are explored within a scientific framework. Learning is direct and experiential as well. Next, a 9-day (66 h) Summer Intensive Practicum (or 8-week MBSR class with additional instruction totally 70 h) is required that invites the future teacher to live inside the experience of a participant-observer while maintaining a practitioner perspective. The trainee is immersed in the CFM approach to teaching MBSR by working in small and large groups with senior teachers. Required reading is distributed prior to taking the course. Learners practise teaching each other and are provided with feedback. The third step is the Teacher Development Intensive that is open to those who have experience teaching MBSR or have a firm foundation in meditative practice and a strong professional background. This 8-day (92 h) training is interactive and demanding. Teacher skills mentioned above are reinforced. The teacher's intention for teaching and integrity are explored. Refining language usage is highlighted. Certification may be sought by preparing a comprehensive portfolio which includes DVDs showing the teacher in action, letters from patients and colleagues supporting the teacher's skills, materials developed for teaching and a list of all the classes taught. Only those having taught at least four MBSR courses and having had supervision are encouraged to apply. Finally, there is an apprentice programme in which co-teaching and coaching is provided. Not only is this an extensive undertaking that requires full commitment, it is an expensive route in terms of time and money. One of the authors (PLD) became certified 9 years after the 7-day MBSR residential, having taught 27 courses before submitting her portfolio.

7.3.2   Bangor, Exeter and Oxford Universities

Since Mindfulness-Based Cognitive Therapy (MBCT) is recognised by the UK government's National Institute for Health and Clinical Excellence and is recommended by the National Health Service, an urgent need to train therapists qualified to offer the programme as well as other mindfulness-based interventions has been recognised. Crane et al. [10] describe and discuss developments in the United Kingdom where three universities (Bangor, Exeter and Oxford) have teacher training programmes, some at the masters' level. They subdivide training into four phases: foundational, basic teacher, early teacher, advanced and continuing professional development. Similar to MBSR teacher training, the first step is to take a course (MBCT or MBSR). For the second step, regular meditation practice and partaking in retreats are requisite; for those who will teach MBCT, experience in Cognitive Behavioural Therapy is necessary. Since MBCT was originally conceived to prevent relapse in patients with recurrent clinical depression, this approach is clinical in nature, so it is important the future teachers understand the nature of human suffering and specific patient vulnerabilities (e.g. cognitive distortions in depressed patients). Trainees learn the theories and review research underlying the programme as well as its intention, structure and organisation. Future teachers practise among each other and receive supervision. For advanced training, students continue with supervision while teaching courses. Opportunities to reflect and exchange their experiences are extended to learners. Given that work is aimed more towards mental health professionals, it may interest a subset of future teachers of Mindful Medical Practice (notably psychiatrists and psychologists) and thus will not be elaborated upon here. What is relevant in Crane et al.'s [10, 11] work is teacher assessment. For example, a tool has been developed whereby six domains essential to teaching are rated; these are coverage, pacing and organisation of session curriculum, relationship skills, embodiment of mindfulness, guiding mindfulness practices, conveying course themes through interactive inquiry and didactic teaching and the management of the group learning environment. The tool aims to measure integrity in three areas: teacher competence, level of adherence (i.e. programme fidelity) and differentiation (excludes elements that do not belong in the programme).

7.3.3   University of Rochester School of Medicine and Dentistry

Led by Drs. Epstein and Krasner and their colleagues, the University of Rochester School of Medicine and Dentistry offer, twice a year, an accredited 4–5-day residential workshop to 'Train the Trainers'; most participants are physicians. One of the authors (PLD) attended two workshops; the first given in 2010 was entitled, 'Promoting

Mindful Practice in Medical Education'; the second given in 2015 was entitled, 'Mindful Practice Advanced Workshop: Enhancing Quality of Care, Quality of Caring and Resilience'.

The learning objectives of the 2010 workshop were:

- Incorporate mindful curricula into undergraduate, graduate and continuing education programmes.
- Lead experiential exercises that involve meditation, mindfulness, self-awareness exercises, narrative writing, group discussion and didactic material.
- Enhance one's own capacity for self-awareness and self-monitoring, including attentive observation, curiosity, informed flexibility and presence.

The themes covered were:

- Cognition – how doctors notice, perceive and think
- Errors – how and why we make errors, how to prevent them and disclosure/apology once they occur
- Burnout and well-being – how to recognise burnout and how to enhance well-being, work/home balance
- Self-monitoring – how we know how we are doing, automatic and deliberative processing, how we know when to slow down
- Challenges to professionalism – attraction to patients, monetary incentives, conflict, pressure to prescribe, boundaries, limits

The workshop was balanced between experiential discovery and learning how to teach the material. Meditation, narrative writing, Appreciative Inquiry, small and large group discussions pertaining to the experiences and didactic material were spread across the days. Learners were given teaching materials: PowerPoint presentations, articles and CDs to work with so that they could move directly into teaching following the workshop. They were invited to determine what would work best in their own settings, be it with medical students, residents or practising physicians. It opened vistas to variations such as offering half-day, full day and weekend workshops. Much like the training for MBSR, future teachers were encouraged to engage in contemplative practice so that their teaching naturally arises from it. This experience shows that the 8-week MBSR format is one among other formats for teaching mindfulness.

The advanced workshop in 2015 attracted clinicians and educators who were engaged in Mindful Practice in various ways; many were returning for reasons such as to learn new skills, to exchange with others who were already doing this work, to reconnect with like-minded/hearted clinicians or simply to support their own practice. One of the authors who attended (PLD) was interested in how these experts were training the teachers. From the first evening, small groups were formed and reformed to introduce concepts (such as presence) and people to one another through dialogue. Throughout the week space was provided for participants to interact, formally in 'affinity groups' who met six separate times, read and explored poems together with a minimum of instruction. Given the relatively large size of the group (46), the affinity groups (of 6 participants) encouraged people to get to know one another. Informal meeting was promoted during 12 healthy meals, with the workshop leaders sitting among the others. Thus, a warm atmosphere for being together was offered; this 'container' made it 'safe' for deep reflection and sharing to occur.

Similar to the 2010 workshop, teaching tools, such as narrative medicine and Appreciative Inquiry, were interwoven in large group settings and then practised in four medium-sized groups that were facilitated by one of the faculty members leading the workshop. For those who had never taught meditation, they were given an opportunity to do this and receive feedback. In the mid-size groups, participants role-played Appreciative Inquiry so as to hone this skill. DVDs were viewed as springboards for discussions; music as a metaphor for engaging with others. A lending library was available for those who wished to deepen their knowledge. CDs of all the teachings were provided.

Informal practice was encouraged. Trainees were asked to notice their surroundings, observe how they interact with others and explore how their bodies move through space. Midway through the week, the group entered a silent period from 5:30 PM, including a silent supper, through to the end of the morning. Along with the daily 6:30–7:30 AM sitting and walking meditation in the Zendo (meditation hall), the important point that one needs to have a personal practice to teach this material was clearly made.

Intriguingly, when the group was ending and debriefing the week together, a physician from South America made a comment that gave pause to all. She said, hoping the translation from Spanish to English was correct, 'You taught nothing and I learned so much'. The faculty members interpreted this statement as the highest form of a complement. They understood that their job as teachers was to lead the learners to discover for themselves what they were ready to incorporate in their work and lives.

7.3.4   *Monash University Faculty of Medicine, Nursing and Health Sciences*

As coordinator of mindfulness programmes at Monash University, one of the authors (CSH) convenes and is responsible for tutor employment and training for the mindfulness programmes in the medical faculty. The main prerequisites are that potential tutors are health professionals who maintain a personal and professional experience with and commitment to mindfulness and that they are experienced in group work. The personal commitment to mindfulness is particularly important because much of the teaching of mindfulness occurs via modelling, not merely by engaging with it on a theoretical level. All tutors are interviewed about their experience and motivation prior to being engaged as tutors.

While a few are faculty members, most teach as casual tutors and come from their practices or other professional engagements. Many of them will also subsequently tutor in other Monash faculties which also have embedded mindfulness curriculum such as physiotherapy, IT and pharmacy.

Tutor training into the Monash University medical curriculum can take various forms. Many will have already completed extensive training outside of Monash University in MBSR or MBCT or other generic mindfulness courses provided at the university. If they have been previously using mindfulness professionally, then these tutors will undergo a 3 h tutor orientation to the Monash medical student mindfulness programme followed by pre-readings and tutor notes. Even so, if they are to be involved for the first time, then they will be mentored by sitting in with and observing an experienced tutor so that they observe how the programme is run before they take it themselves. This acquaints them not only with the tutorial content but also the teaching style we wish them to adopt.

For prospective tutors who are relatively new to mindfulness but have a growing interest in it then, firstly, they will be encouraged to take basic mindfulness training themselves. Next, they are invited to do a train-the-trainer programme which takes place for over four 90 min sessions. The topics for the 4 weeks are:

- Involving the individual or group, including:

    (a) The importance of personal practice for the mindfulness teacher
    (b) Modelling an introduction to mindfulness in the first tutorial

        1. Exploring the cost of being unmindful
        2. Rendering mindfulness relevant: expressing its application in terms of what is important to the individual or group (study, stress, coping with emotions, sleep)
        3. Introducing mindfulness in simple, familiar and practical terms
        4. Engaging students with questions, not statements to open inquiry
        5. Encouraging experimentation and being non-judgmental

    (c) Reflecting on the introduction and what was noticed or learned

- Teaching mindfulness meditation

    (a) Introducing the meditation practice including

        1. Linking formal practice to cultivating awareness in daily life
        2. Seeing it as an experiment
        3. Reinforcing that personal practice is voluntary for the students
        4. No pressure about getting it right or wrong, just learning from experience

    (b) Leading the practice – practise what you teach

        1. Pacing, tone of voice, attitude of acceptance
        2. Finishing the practice and debriefing student experience
        3. No failing – inviting exploration

    (c) Encouraging home practice – how long and how often?

        1. Full stops (5 min twice a day) and frequent commas (short practices of 15–60 s) to punctuate the day
        2. Guided or not guided? Which is best?

    3. How to debrief home practice. Was it practised at home during the week? If so, what was discovered? If not, what were the barriers to practising mindfulness meditation?

- Debriefing mindfully – mindful inquiry

    (a) Modelling the debriefing process by debriefing the tutors' weekly formal and informal practice of mindfulness
    (b) Reflecting on the debriefing process
    (c) Examining the importance of mindful inquiry:

        1. Openness
        2. Curiosity
        3. Acceptance
        4. Learning trumps apparent 'success' and 'failure'

    (d) Introducing the 'big 4' cognitive practices for exploration:

        1. Perception
        2. Letting go (non-attachment)
        3. Acceptance
        4. Presence of mind

- Cognitive practices, course structure and teaching a series of 'mindfulness experiments'

    (a) Debriefing the tutors' application of the cognitive aspects in their own life

        1. Further reflection of the debriefing process

    (b) Modelling mindfulness experiments

        1. Multitasking
        2. Mindful communication
        3. Dealing with distractor influence
        4. Mindful eating

    (c) Discussing course structure and how to focus on relevant objectives
    (d) Reviewing questions and answers

If all proceeds well and they are accumulating personal and professional experience in mindfulness, then the following year they will be invited to sit in with an experienced tutor before being given the opportunity to teach the next year.

7.4 Supervision and Mentorship

Fledgling mindfulness teachers are like apprentices. They will master their trade by working with masters who take it upon themselves to transmit the knowledge and know-how of teaching mindfulness honed through years of experience and reflection.

The relationship between the supervisor and supervisee is unique because it transpires within the space of awareness of the self, the other and the context. The supervisor needs to be congruent and respectful of the supervisee's trajectory, meeting him/her where she/he is. For example, 'Is this the first class the new teacher has ever taught? How long has she/he been practising body-mind exercises, such as yoga, him- or herself? Is this person in a work environment that is inherently stressful (e.g. a resident in a children's hospital)?' As described in Dobkin and Laliberté [12], the characteristics of a mindful clinical teacher apply to being a mindful supervisor. The teacher-student relationship is vital: it needs to be respectful, collaborative in nature, entail an emotional investment and recognise the inherent reciprocal nature of the process. Keeping in mind that a supervisor is also a model, she/he needs to, as best they are able, embody the characteristics of mindfulness mentioned earlier in this chapter (e.g. open and curious, patient), clarify his/her intentions for supervising and stay attuned to the present moment while interacting with the teacher in training. Thus, there is more than content to cover when supervising. How one is with the trainee is as important as what is said and done.

The supervisor primes him/herself by reflecting on the purpose of the work. Asking, 'What is my intention?' is a good way to start. Next, it is imperative to be available in the true sense of the word: mentally, emotionally and within a time and place where the exchange takes place. The supervisor invites curiosity by asking reflective questions about relevant aspects of the teaching experience such as, 'While you were teaching did you notice the rhythm of your own breath? Did it change when you felt rushed or apprehensive? How did you respond to that? Did you notice where your attention went while you were conversing with the students about their experience? Did you notice what reactions arose when a student expressed ambivalence about practising mindfulness? If so, how did you respond to your own reaction and to the student? What was the effect of that response?' This encourages the supervisee to stay alert while teaching. Ideally if such experiences are debriefed in a non-judgmental way, it invites the supervisee to take the same attitude towards their own experience.

The supervisor may also choose to teach by thinking out loud, i.e. making mental processes transparent. She/he may say something like, 'While I was watching the DVD of your first class I noticed my thoughts return to what my supervisor told me when I taught my first class. I too felt torn between the course requirements and time constraints. My supervisor emphasized the need to balance the structure of the curriculum with flexibility such that I could respond to the moment'. Or, perhaps the supervisee noticed an internal dialogue with themselves like, 'What's wrong with me? My mind keeps wandering off. I should be better than this? How can I teach it if I can't even practice it?' Giving voice to such internal dialogues makes them more recognisable and may soften the criticism. Equally as important, the supervisor practises presence with the supervisee such that the latter feels heard, understood and respected. The conscious use of language that is not judgmental or critical is indispensable as this will enable the supervisee to integrate the feedback without being humiliated or discouraged. Following the exchange the supervisor can reflect on the encounter afterwards as part of his/her own learning process. When humour peppers the exchange the experience is more agreeable.

Supervision may be based on audiotapes, DVDs of sessions, journal entries and verbal reports. Issues related to confidentiality and boundaries need to be clarified up front and supervision formats should be agreed upon before embarking on this endeavour. Starting with a short meditation practice can set the stage for how this type of teaching differs from most, with both parties committing to being mindful throughout the exchange. Rather than focus exclusively on content, the supervisor and supervisee draw from their direct experiences while in reflection and dialogue together. Open-ended questions during inquiry are more likely to facilitate the learning process. The supervisor, recalling the notion of common humanity, is encouraged to be open to learning from the exchange as well.

Evans et al. [13] proposed a framework for supervision of MBSR and MBCT teachers. It consists of circles within circles with the outer circle being the 'container of mindfulness', i.e. staying aware while supervising. The authors state that 'the whole of teaching/training process is mindfulness-based'. Supervisors' embodied presence, integrity and intentions are found within this outer circle. There is a bidirectional flow between the 'supervision space' (the inner circle) which includes mutual inquiry, present moment focus, integration and (a) teaching skills, (b) personal practice/process, (c) people in the group and (d) theory/understanding. These four areas (a–d) are the middle circles that constitute the content and themes of supervision.

7.5   The Ethical Space for Training Teachers

McCowen's call to place teacher training within an ethical view is radical in that it takes the focus off the individual and moves it towards teacher development within the context of the gathering. A teacher is seen as a 'multi-being'. Rather than put singular emphasis on the teacher's personal meditation practice, attendance at retreats, etc., how the teacher is in relation to others in the room is crucial to being a good-enough teacher. He states, 'To develop as a teacher is to incorporate the potentials generated through co-creation of mindfulness' [6] (p. 207). Skills are not mastered in isolation, as if the teacher must change him/herself or attain a level of wisdom through years of meditation. It is helpful to be part of mindfulness teaching communities where one can 'steep oneself in the practice of pedagogy' [6] (p. 211). Of course, if the mindfulness teacher is also a clinician who uses mindfulness in their daily work, then this makes the job easier as they are constantly being reminded about it. As professionals training other professionals who will encounter thousands of patients over decades of medical practice, it is our responsibility to ensure that training is carried out with the intention to relieve suffering in whatever form it takes.

References

1. France A. The crime of Sylvestre Bonnard (L. Hearn, trans). Vol. 1 of The Works of Anatole France; Gabriel Wells, Paris France. 1924. Part 2, Chapter 4, 6 June 1860. p. 198.
2. McCowen D, Reibel D, Micozzi MS. Teaching mindfulness: a practical guide for clinicians and educators. New York: Springer; 2011.
3. Edmondson AC, Bohmer R, Pisano GP. Speeding up team learning. Harv Bus Rev. 2001; 79(9):125–34.
4. Van Aalderen JR, Breukers WJ, Reuzel RPB, Speckens AEM. The role of the teacher in mindfulness-based approaches: a qualitative approach. Mindfulness. 2014;5:170–8.
5. Dobkin PL, Isnard-Bagnis C, Spodenkiewicz M. Being human in medicine: beyond hierarchy. Int J Whole Person Care. 2015;2(1):38–49.
6. McCowen D. The ethical space of mindfulness in clinical practice. London: Jessica Kingsley Publishers; 2013.
7. Crane RS, Stanley S, Rooney M, Bartley T, Coper L, Mardula J. Disciplined improvisation: characteristics of inquiry in mindfulness-based teaching. Mindfulness. 2014. doi:10.1007/s12671-014-0361-8.
8. Epstein RM. Just being. West J Med. 2001;174:63–5.
9. Hickman S, Ucok O, Krasner M. Workshop: rhetoric, rhythm and the rest between two beats: conversation analysis as a profound teaching in mindfulness. 2008 Integrating Mindfulness-Based Interventions into Medicine, Health Care and the Larger Society. The 6th Annual Conference for Clinicians, Researchers and Educators. Worcester. 2008
10. Crane RS, Kuyken W, Hastings RP, Rothwell N, Williams JM. Training teachers to deliver mindfulness-based interventions: learning from the UK experience. Mindfulness. 2010; 1(2):74–86.
11. Crane RS, Eames C, Kuyken W, Hastings RP, Mark JG, Bartley WT, et al. Development and validation of the mindfulness-based interventions – teaching assessment criteria (MBI:TAC). Assessment. 2013;20(6):681–8.
12. Dobkin PL, Laliberté V. Being a mindful clinical teacher: can mindfulness enhance education in a clinical setting? Med Teach. 2014;36(4):347–52. doi:10.3109/0142159X.2014.887834.
13. Evans A, Crane R, Cooper L, Mardula J, Wilks J, Surawy C, et al. A framework for supervision for mindfulness-based teachers: a space for embodied mutual inquiry. Mindfulness. 2014. doi:10.1007/s12671-014-0292-4. DOI 10.1007/s12671-014-0292-4, published online March 23, 2014.

Chapter 8
Future Directions, Culture and Caveats for Mindfulness in Medical Settings

8.1 Leadership

Although the emphasis in most research examined in this book has been on the individual within medical educational and work settings, enhancing the individual's ability to personally manage demanding environments should not be seen in isolation from the need to reform the environments within which the individual learns and works [1]. The workplace culture within which medical students are educated and junior doctors are trained can be unsupportive and even abusive. This raises the need for mindful leadership in developing environments and cultures that foster health professionals' learning, well-being and performance. There is evidence that mindfulness-based workplace programmes help to build resilience and reduce frustration even in unsupportive and controlling work environments [2], but some have raised legitimate concerns that mindfulness-based workplace interventions aimed at enhancing individual performance and resilience in dysfunctional work environments could make it easy to ignore the need for systemic or cultural change and lead to further abuse of workers [3].

The work done thus far has stimulated interest in the development of mindful attributes among medical leaders. These include enhancing resilience, empathy, attentive communication and sound decision-making while under pressure [4, 5]. Knowledge reviewed in Chap. 2 pertaining to improved mental health, communication, emotional intelligence and neuroscience point to mindfulness as being a means for enhancing leadership.

There are multiple reports of interventions successfully incorporating mindfulness as a way of improving the culture of the workplace in medical settings, but these have generally not been subjected to rigorous evaluation [6]. One randomised study of the effect of mindfulness with corporate senior managers found enhanced participants' self-perception of leadership skills as a bundle of all five skills, with three out of five individual skills – inspiring a shared vision, demonstrating moral intelligence and encouraging the heart/motivating – changing most significantly [7].

© Springer International Publishing Switzerland 2016
P.L. Dobkin, C.S. Hassed, *Mindful Medical Practitioners*,
DOI 10.1007/978-3-319-31066-4_8

A mindfulness programme run for university staff by Atkins et al. demonstrated increased self-rated performance, improved well-being, improved eudaimonic well-being (meaningfulness), increase in two subscales of work engagement (vigour and dedication), increased authenticity (self-awareness, authentic behaviour, open relationships) and increased satisfaction with life. These improvements were sustained at 6-month follow-up [8]. Mindfulness has also been found to reduce negative affect in leaders which is one significant source of stress and poor performance [9]. Faculty facilitators who were trained in a mind-body medicine course which included mindfulness training scored significantly lower on perceived stress and higher on mindfulness compared with controls [10]. Qualitative analysis revealed central themes including professional identity (subthemes of communication, connections and community, empathy and active listening and self-confidence), self-care and mindful awareness. Mindful leadership programmes for medical students have also been found to increase cooperation and team-based communication [11].

The impact of mindfulness on leadership effectiveness in a health-care setting was reported by Wasylkiw et al. [12]. The approach was unique in that mid-level health-care managers participated in an intensive weekend retreat and compared to a control group that did not. Self-report and co-workers' reports were gathered, and the retreat participants were interviewed 4–8 weeks later to determine if they were integrating what they learned in their work settings. Retreat participants were more mindful, less stressed and more effective as leaders after the course. 'Informants' in their work setting corroborated these leadership changes in the extent the participants in the retreat were open with others (i.e. transparent) and solicited others' viewpoints. While the interview data were rich in descriptions of how mindfulness was applied at work, the managers were unable to maintain formal meditation practices in a chaotic environment that did not value self-care or provide time or space for developing resilience.

8.2   Changing the Culture of Medicine: Two Model Programmes

Considering widespread criticism of the oftentimes abusive medical culture within which medical students and junior doctors are trained [13], this is certainly fertile ground for new programmes and research. Herein we briefly highlight two model programmes that have taken on this challenge: one in a medical school setting and the other within a hospital and community care setting.

8.2.1   Indiana University School of Medicine

Williamson et al. [14] describe how, beginning in 2003, the Indiana University School of Medicine faced the enormous challenge of changing the medical school culture with courage and determination over a 4-year period. They called this endeavour the Relationship-Centred Care Initiative. The leadership group adopted an 'emergent design' strategy that involved pursuing change but allowing the specific path of implementation emerges through collaboration between project leaders and members of the organisation [15]. It is described as maintaining a willingness to 'not know', identifying 'kindred spirits' who share visions and values and trusting that one thing naturally leads to the next. Each step depends on the outcome of the previous step, who had been engaged and what new ideas and opportunities arose. They assembled a formation team with six members (insiders and consultants) who brought unique talents and experiences to the group such that they would complement each other in their tasks. They served as the stewards of the entire project. Early on they met with senior leaders – the dean and executive associate deans to exchange ideas and reflect on their work. This support from the top was critical to their overall success.

A discovery team (with 12 members, including administrative leaders, physicians, nurses, patent advocates, to name a few) conducted 80 Appreciative Inquiry interviews to determine what was going well within their institution. Students, residents and alumni were included in this process. Four themes were identified:

- Believing in the capacity of people to learn and grow: trusting them to take on a higher level of responsibility
- Connectedness: between students and teachers, patients and clinicians, members of interdisciplinary health-care teams, research collaborators, scientists and clinicians and members of various departments and institutions
- Passion for one's work
- 'Wonderment' of medicine

When these results were presented in an open forum, others joined to participate in the project.

Two programmes, Courage to Lead (four seasonal retreats for three consecutive years) and Internal Change Agent (five-session, 20 h skill development) enabled those who volunteered to learn more about fostering positive changes. Their work was based on the premise that change takes place one person at a time and from the inside out – for the person and the organisation.

Monthly peer-coaching meetings took place so that they could share their goals and practices with committees such as Professional Standards, Academic Standards and Teacher-Learner Advocacy.

External consultants met with a network of department chairs, programme directors, nurse researchers, administrators, staff, students, residents and other school leaders to invite participation and support. Student and resident engagement teams surfaced from this effort. They met bimonthly and shared stories about relationship-centred practices and were coached within a safe setting. Not surprisingly this was harder to do with residents due to their work demands and lack of control over their schedules; thus, this aspect of the project was less successful.

Given that the institution had sites across the state, they travelled and conducted videoconferences. They secured funding and focused on external dissemination through a National Immersion Conference. They shared data on participation in activities, direct observations about change patterns (e.g. at the individual and organ-isational levels) and new institutional developments. For example, one unplanned change was the project's influence on medical student admissions process. Relationship-centred values were assessed as part of the admission interviews. An independent evaluator assessed the project outcomes as well; changes were seen in performance reviews, how meetings were conducted and staff communications. Student survey results on satisfaction with the quality of their medical education increased over the 4-year period.

The lessons learned were:

- Changing global patterns of relating in what they call organisational culture involves changes in the local patterns of everyday interactions.
- The changes in the medical school included both 'top-down' and 'bottom-up' processes.
- Positive patterns were reinforced through circles of reciprocal influence.
- Beliefs and expectations influence change: without hope that change is possible and without expectations that people will do their best if given the chance, people and institutions will rest stuck in old, dysfunctional patterns.
- The emergent design was deemed a successful strategy.

8.2.2   Discovering Resilience: A Community Partnership to Enhance Workplace Wellness in Health Care - Andrea Frolic [16]

An inter-professional, multi-institutional partnership to promote resilience through mindful practices was initiated by a small grass-roots group of health-care practitio-ners at Hamilton Health Sciences in Hamilton, Canada, in 2009. They called them-selves the Discovering Resilience Leadership Team (DRLT)[1] as they aimed to discover and implement evidence-based interventions to support health professionals to cope with vicarious trauma, mounting financial pressures and organisational change while providing compassionate care to their patients and families; their ulti-mate goal was to transform the hospital's culture to become more person centred.

They found an ally in the Program for Faculty Development in the Faculty of Health Sciences at McMaster University, who agreed to provide organisational sup-port for a pilot mindfulness course. The DRLT found mentors and teachers to support

[1] Thanks to the founding members of the Discovering Resilience Leadership Team at Hamilton Health Sciences (2009–2015): Andrea Frolic (Director, Office of Clinical & Organizational Ethics), Elaine Principi (Chief of inter-professional practice), Valerie Spironello (social worker) and Dr. Alan Taniguchi (palliative care physician). Partner members of the DRLT (2013–2015): Dr. Ken Burgess (family physician), Savinna Frederiksen (social worker), Dr. Michael Vesselago (family physician) and Joyce Zazulak (family physician). Deep gratitude extended to Dr. Denise Marshall and Dr. Anne Wong, Assistant Deans of the McMaster Program for Faculty Development, and the support of their staff Annette Sciarra and Elda DiCroce for their expert administration.

the development of a course that would meet the distinctive needs and context of health-care providers; this first course was entitled 'Developing Resilience through Applied Mindfulness', structured as four weekend modules, each with a different focus (e.g. the foundations of mindfulness, neuroscience and the application of mindfulness in education and health care). After this successful pilot, additional courses were added to the curriculum to support the integration of mindfulness into personal/professional life for health-care professionals/faculty. These included a traditional MBSR course, as well as novel courses, including a Transforming Compassion Fatigue workshop, Narrative Medicine workshops and a Mindful Communication course modelled on a curriculum from the University of Rochester. The courses offered are evidence-based and adapted to the reality of the health-care setting, as described in Chap. 6.

For the DRLT, mindfulness is viewed as whole person education that focuses on:

- The need to develop a relationship with suffering
- The power of compassion to transform relationships
- Knowledge based on neuroscience
- The importance of experiential learning over time (via meditation practices)
- Recognition that the personal and professional are intrinsically linked
- Self-care as essential to care for others
- An emphasis on the ethical dimensions of mindfulness through practices that promote value-based behaviour (like setting intentions)

From the beginning the DRLT was committed to providing high-quality courses with well-qualified teachers. They created a teacher mentorship programme to support the development of new mindfulness teachers. Their standards are consistent with those described in Chap. 7.

In 2013 Hamilton Health Sciences and St. Joseph's Healthcare Hamilton created a partnership through a Healthy Work Environment Partnership and Innovation Fund Grant from the Ontario Ministry of Health and Long Term Care. The goal was to develop expertise in creating and delivering mindfulness courses to front-line workers and measuring outcomes. An interdisciplinary research team was assembled with colleagues from McMaster University (including researchers in psychology, anthropology and rehabilitation science) to plan data collection and analyses. Preliminary results were published in a paper by Moll et al. [17] entitled, 'Investing in Compassion: Exploring mindfulness as a strategy to enhance interpersonal relationships in health care practice'. The team employed a mixed-method, non-randomised intervention study to track the impact of MBSR with 164 employees in the two participating hospitals. Recruitment strategies used were 'lunch and learn' sessions, email flyers, staff newsletters and reaching out to employees in high-stress positions as well as those in clinical leadership jobs. Two focus groups were conducted 1 year later with 12 participants (5 managers and 6 clinicians). Overall, there were significant changes in:

- Improved empathetic concern, perspective taking (cognitive aspects of empathy)
- Decreases in emotional exhaustion and depersonalisation (burnout characteristics)

- Descriptions of being able to listen better, being more tolerant and compassionate
- Decreases in emotional reactivity and personal distress
- Improved interactions with colleagues, patients and family
- Better skills at managing conflict

These positive results were presented to policymakers within Hamilton Health Sciences and St. Joseph's Healthcare Hamilton, as well as to members of two large primary care groups, McMaster Family Health Team and Hamilton Family Health Team. Representatives of these organisations joined the DRLT and successfully advocated to forge a multi-institutional partnership to offer mindfulness-based interventions to health-care staff/physicians/faculty at a subsidised rate through the McMaster Program for Faculty Development. Impressively, in their first 6 years, over 600 health-care professionals in Hamilton participated in a mindfulness course. Leadership engagement has been key to the success of this initiative, specifically, providing leaders with a direct, personal experience of mindfulness while connecting mindfulness to both scientific evidence and organisational strategic priorities.

The DRLT has also developed structures and supports to help course graduates sustain and integrate mindfulness practice in the workplace. A Professional 'Sangha' (a spiritual community) was formed for course graduates to gather monthly to meditate together, with facilitators from the community leading practices on a donation basis. Hamilton Health Sciences created a page within their staff wellness site (www.shinehhs.ca/get-healthy/be-mindful) specifically dedicated to educating staff about mindfulness and promoting hospital-based mindfulness resources. A Mindfulness for Lunch toolkit was developed within the hospitals to encourage meditation practice in the workplace. In addition, the Ministry of Health and Long Term Care grant provided seed money for a community-based mindfulness group and website (www.mindfulnesshamilton.ca) to connect the people of Hamilton with mindfulness resources. Mindfulness Hamilton now offers weekly meditation groups and mindfulness retreats for the community.

From the beginning, the DRLT understood that culture change requires a social movement. So they gathered a group of people who shared common values and a commitment to champion change from within. Their common goal is to enhance the quality of care and teaching by empowering caregivers and faculty to listen to and care for themselves. Their common values are:

- Inter-professional collaboration
- Peace as the common root
- Reflective emergence (i.e. reflecting and adjusting with experience)
- Secular yet sacred (i.e. promoting mindfulness as a secular practice yet honouring its sacred dimensions)
- Diversity not dogma (i.e. recognising the myriad ways mindfulness can be practised to promote personal and cultural change)

These common values have emboldened the DRLT to sustain and grow its counter-cultural grass-roots movement in the face of scepticism, overt opposition and resource scarcity. Today, mindfulness is being integrated into leadership meetings, patient care and teamwork across partner organisations, and graduates are reporting remarkable enhancement of their well-being at work and at home.

Kearsley and Youngson [18] underscore the need for work being carried out by Frolic and her colleagues in their paper on the compassionate hospital. This is defined as a health-care facility whose staff has a deep awareness of, and responds to, the suffering that arises from illness. The overlapping characteristics of a compassionate hospital are the presence of a healing environment, a sense of connection between people (staff, staff and patients, staff and the community) and a sense of purpose and direction. Leadership is vital to the cultural change needed for such a place to be more than an ideal or dream. Mindfulness plays the role of contributing to the inner resources needed, along with reflection, creativity, self-awareness and resilience that would help reintegrate a humane environment that sustains those who serve others with the intention to reduce their suffering.

8.3   Is Mindfulness a Panacea?

With all the applications currently offered, the many positive findings coming to light and an increasingly large and enthusiastic number of advocates, mindfulness could easily be considered as a panacea. To some extent that may be a legitimate view in that mindfulness is an innate ability with many different applications and demonstrated benefits. There are, nonetheless, legitimate concerns about thinking it is a cure all. The fact that becoming mindful *could* be valuable for someone doesn't mean that he or she *will* benefit by practising it. For example:

- Just as a person may know that physical exercise is good for health, and they understand its benefits, they may not make the effort to do it. Similarly, one challenge underlying mindfulness is knowing how to assist a person, particularly one who is not distressed, to overcome the inertia preventing him from applying mindfulness.
- A person may be poorly taught by an inexperienced or misinformed teacher of mindfulness. This is an increasing concern as many professionals receive limited mindfulness training before teaching it to others, especially when that training is divorced from mindfulness' philosophical and ethical foundation.
- It may be difficult for a person to learn mindfulness in the presence of significant and unpleasant experiences such as in major anxiety and depression or severe pain. The teacher needs to be very experienced with the particular condition(s) and know how to teach mindfulness effectively in such situations. For example, rebound anxiety can occur (much like rebound insomnia after stopping medications); while this is not an adverse event per se, a clinician needs to offer skilful care and guidance in how to work with such experiences so that they do not escalate and that insight can arise.
- A person could be thrust into a mindfulness programme without their full agreement. If the person perceives mindfulness as being imposed upon him or her, this

will be counterproductive. It is vital to respect a person's preferences and inclinations. For some, simply cultivating an appreciation of the impact of 'unmindfulness' may be an adequate first step. Sometimes the skilful teaching of mindfulness means not to teach it until a person is ready. This issue is germane when mindfulness is included in core medical curriculum. Each person has the freedom to choose whether to practise it in their personal life.

• Although uncommon, adverse events may occur. There are anecdotal reports of people with a history of psychosis having negative experiences, particularly when meditating intensively (e.g. during a week-long silent retreat). Mindfulness meditation is contraindicated for acute psychosis. A person who experiences significant rebound anxiety or has a past history of abuse may have their symptoms magnified. Uncomfortable as it may be, this is not necessarily an adverse event if the person is carefully guided in how to work with such experiences. Thus, a clinician should assess the risk before including a person in a meditation programme. Moreover, it is not recommended for a person who is actively abusing substances.

These caveats provide a case for the skilful teaching of mindfulness: experienced practitioners teaching it in the right context, with the right language, the right way, at the right time and at the right pace.

8.4   Beware of 'McMindfulness'

Purser and Loy [3] caution about mindfulness going mainstream to the extent that its essence is lost. Its commercialisation has the potential to divorce it from its philosophical roots, which can be found in Buddhism and other wisdom traditions, such that the intention to be compassionate and relieve suffering is forgotten. Madhavin et al. [19] reviewed and evaluated 560 telephone apps finding only 23 met their criteria – including education and training. Most were timers, reminders or only guided meditations; very few had high ratings. The authors pointed out that mindfulness is much more than meditation, a breathing technique or relaxation exercise. Headspace scored highest (4/5) on a scale that included engagement, functionality, visual appeal, information quality and subjective quality as it integrated community support as well. One app entitled 'OMG I can meditate' is an example of a commercialised app that would not meet the authors' standards. On their website one finds, 'We can make meditation a no brainer', along with, 'perform better' and promises that meditation is 'Simple. Enjoyable. Effective' and 'Think of it as a hug for your mind'.

When the ethical basis of mindfulness is overlooked or neglected, then the potential for exploitation is present. Apparently the media has missed the point that there can be 'right mindfulness' and 'wrong mindfulness'. 'Right' means wise and skilful with an explicit intention to care for others and to do no harm, and 'wrong' is based on selfish motivation which ignores the well-being of others. For a more in-depth discussion of these issues, the reader is referred to Monteiro et al. [20]. The commercialisation of something that is so popular is not surprising. It is not in itself a fault with mindfulness per se but is a sign of its success and the widespread longing for something meaningful. Even so, the skill, motivation and authenticity of mindfulness teachers may be corrupted by success and this remains a concern.

As HH the Dalaï Lama teaches [21], first examine your intention. There are three orientations towards work: a *job* provides income, a *career* allows for advancement and success, and a *calling* involves meaningful work that serves a higher purpose such as social good and the welfare of others. Ask yourself, 'Am I motivated to foster wellness in myself so that I may serve others?' We need to remember, and to remind medical students and residents, this is the core reason why we practise the art and science of medicine.

References

1. Dobkin PL, Hutchinson TA. Primary prevention for future doctors: promoting well-being in trainees. Med Educ. 2010;44(3):224–6.
2. Schultz PP, Ryan RM, Niemiec CP, Legate N, Williams GC. Mindfulness, work climate, and psychological need satisfaction in employee well-being. Mindfulness. 2015;6(5):971–85. doi:10.1007/s12671-014-0338-7.
3. Purser R, Loy D. Beyond McMindfulness. The Huffington Post Australia [Internet]. 2013 [cited 2015 Nov 24]. Available from: http://www.huffingtonpost.com/ron-purser/beyond-mcmindfulness_b_3519289.html?ir=Australia.
4. Wicks RJ, Buck TC. Riding the dragon: enhancing resilient leadership and sensible self-care in the healthcare executive. Front Health Serv Manag. 2013;30(2):3–13.
5. Kelley-Patterson D. What kind of leadership does integrated care need? Lond J Prim Care (Abingdon). 2012;5(1):3–7.
6. Egener B, McDonald W, Rosof B, Gullen D. Perspective: organizational professionalism: relevant competencies and behaviors. Acad Med. 2012;87(5):668–74. doi:10.1097/ACM.0b013e31824d4b67.
7. Amar AD, Hlupic V, Tamwatin T. Effect of meditation on self-perception of leadership skills: a controlled group study of CEOs. Acad Manag Proc. 2014;1:14282. doi:10.5465/AMBPP.2014.300.
8. Atkins PWB, Hassed C, Fogliati VJ. Mindfulness improves work engagement, wellbeing and performance in a University setting. In: Burke RJ, Cooper CL, Page KM, editors. Flourishing in life, work, and careers. Individual wellbeing and career experiences. Cheltenham: Edward Elgar Publishing; 2015.
9. Roche M, Haar JM, Luthans F. The role of mindfulness and psychological capital on the well-being of leaders. J Occup Heal Psychol. 2014;19(4):476–89. doi:10.1037/a0037183.
10. Talisman N, Harazduk N, Rush C, Graves K, Haramati A. The impact of mind-body medicine facilitation on affirming and enhancing professional identity in health care professions faculty. Acad Med. 2015;90(6):780–4. doi:10.1097/ACM.0000000000000720.
11. Warde CM, Vermillion M, Uijtdehaage S. A medical student leadership course led to teamwork, advocacy, and mindfulness. Fam Med. 2014;46(6):459–62.
12. Wasylkiw L, Holton J, Azar R, Cook W. The impact of mindfulness on leadership effectiveness in a health care setting: a pilot study. J Heal Org Manag. 2015;29(7):893–911.
13. Allen D, Wainwright M, Mount B, Hutchinson TA. The wounding path to becoming healers: medical students' apprenticeship experiences. Med Teach. 2008;30(3):260–4.
14. Williamson PR, Baldwin DC, Cottingham AH, Frankel R, Inui TS, Litzelman DK, et al. Transforming the professional culture of a medical school from the inside out. In: Suchman AL, Sluyter DJ, Williamson PR, editors. Leading change in healthcare. Transforming organizations

using complexity, positive psychology and relationship-centered care. London: Radcliffe Publishing; 2011.

15. Cottingham AH, Suchman AL, Litzelman DK, Frankel RM, Mossbarger DL, Williamson PR, et al. Enhancing the informal curriculum of a medical school: a case study in organizational culture change. J Gen Inter Med. 2008;23(6):715–22. doi:10.1007/s11606-008-0543-y.
16. Frolic A. Pilgrims together: leveraging community partnerships to enhance workplace resilience. Int J Whole Person Care. 2016 (in press).
17. Moll S, Frolic A, Key B. Investing in compassion: exploring mindfulness as a strategy to enhance interpersonal relationships in health care practice. J Hosp Admin. 2015;4(6):36–45.
18. Kearsley JH, Youngson R. "Tu souffres, cela suffit". The compassionate hospital. J Pall Med. 2012;15(4):457–62.
19. Madhavan M, Kavanagh DJ, Hides L, Stoyanov SR. Review and evaluation of mindfulness-based iPhone apps. JMIR mHealth uHealth. 2015;3(3), e82. doi:10.2196/mhealth.4328.
20. Monteiro LM, Musten RF, Compson J. Traditional and contemporary mindfulness: finding the middle path in the tangle of concerns. Mindfulness. 2015;6:1–13. doi:10.1007/s12671-014-0301-7.
21. Lama D, Cutler HC. The art of happiness at work. New York: Berkley Pub Group; 2003.

Index

© Springer International Publishing Switzerland 2016
P.L. Dobkin, C.S. Hassed, *Mindful Medical Practitioners*,
DOI 10.1007/978-3-319-31066-4

Printed in the United States
By Bookmasters